The Shapes of Memory Loss

Stories, Poems, and Essays from the University of Michigan Medical School and Health System

Nan Barbas

Laura Rice-Oeschger

Cassie Starback

Contributions by Patients, Family Members, and Health Professionals

Disclaimer: Writings in this anthology may include authors' experiences receiving health care or medical treatments. We acknowledge that each author may have had personal and individualized medical experiences and received a variety of recommendations for managing their illness. The contributions to this anthology do not reflect the organizers' or editors' perspectives or recommendations. The content of the writing contained in this anthology is not necessarily representative of state of the art medical knowledge for dementia care.

Cover Design by Kim Cinko

Cover Art: Untitled Watercolor, 2010 by Aviva Robinson, reprinted with permission.

Aviva Robinson's paintings have been shown in numerous galleries and exhibitions throughout Michigan. She has won awards for her art and her philanthropy to the arts. The Detroit Institute of Art, Arts Foundation of Michigan, and Concerned Citizens of the Arts of Michigan are only a few of the organizations for which she has served as board member or committee member. She continues to be a productive painter well into her journey with memory loss.

Published by MPublishing, University of Michigan Library

Content available online at http://openmich/shapes-of-memory-loss

ISBN-13: 978-1-60785-292-6

CONTENTS

Family and friends reflect

Medical students creatively interpret

PREFACE

I recently finished reading Per Petterson's beautiful novel, "Out Stealing Horses," set in Norway, narrated as a reflection by sixty-seven year-old Trond. He reflects on events from the summer when he was fifteen years old that reverberate through the rest of his life. Trond postulates:

"If I just concentrate I can walk into memory's store and find the right shelf with the right film and disappear into it and still feel in my body that ride through the forest with my father."

Petterson's passage beautifully describes the connection that exists between memory and sensation, memory and emotion. I believe that the strength of this type of connection is one explanation for those moments of lucidity that my patients with memory loss or dementia often experience.

We stay connected to our emotional lives and our sensations though, for some, it may be difficult to communicate that connectivity to others. One of the authors of an essay included in this collection becomes reflective when she is told by a woman facing dementia that she intends to write about her illness as "the last thing I write about." The author states this "is interesting since dementia is a disease of memory and personality. In saving your illness for last, your spirit is portrayed…teasing dementia, saying that you will still be able to write your story."

This anthology is a collection of writing that demonstrates the contributors' ability to "walk into memory's store" and to "tease dementia."

We have invited writers to share their experiences with memory loss, to tease dementia. Members of the University of Michigan community submitted poetry, short fiction, journal entries, and narrative essays. Amongst the authors of the pieces included in this collection are patients at the University of Michigan who are experiencing memory loss or cognitive changes due to illnesses such as Alzheimer's disease, strokes, head injuries or other conditions. Some wrote independently of memories of their lives or of their thoughts and feelings about living with changes in their memory or thinking abilities and the effect of those changes on their lives. Some received assistance in expressing these ideas in writing. Other authors included family members and friends who have watched, lived with, cared for, struggled with, or shared laughter about the changes that their husbands, wives, sisters, parents or friends have endured. Professionals who care for patients with cognitive impairment also contributed their reflective thoughts, and a group of doctors-to-be contributed pieces written in the context of interviews conducted with individuals with memory loss.

The inspiration for this project came from our experiences sharing in the journeys of our patients at the Cognitive Disorder Program in the Department of Neurology, and with individuals and groups affected by memory loss who participate in programs at the Michigan Alzheimer's Disease Center and the U-M Silver Club Memory Loss Programs. On a daily basis, we strive to help our patients and their families live the most comfortable and fulfilling lives they can, even as changes confront them. We have drawn on the processes of writing, storytelling, and creative communication. It is in this spirit that this collective, collaborative project, including patients and their extended communities, was undertaken.

We hope readers of this collection enjoy the original, creative, and inspired pieces they will encounter here. We think you will gain a deeper understanding of what it means to live with cognitive changes and memory loss.

Lastly, kudos to the authors. We are awed by their courage to examine the emotions that come with the experience of memory loss due to illness, the immense creativity they demonstrate in recording their emotions in written words, and their extraordinary generosity in sharing their words with others.

Nan Barbas
March, 2013

FOREWORD

"Papa, is that…is that your dad?"

Papa cried. We knew it was so. He had painted an abstract image of his father, richly portrayed in vibrant blue-green watercolors. But he had done it in late-stage Alzheimer's disease, after he had lost his words. Yes, his words. But not his father's memory. Not his own emotional self. Papa was still in there. And he came out in spirit colors for all of us to see and know afresh.

As a neurologist who treats cognitive disorders, I shouldn't have been surprised at his persistent (even new-found) abilities. Research has provided many accounts of incredible expressive potential unleashed in the throes of dementia, traumatic brain injury, stroke, epilepsy, and other neurologic conditions. But I didn't really see it for what it was. My dad was getting his story out. He needed to let us know who he was. He wanted us to feel his elemental fire, still burning in the soul space deep within.

Papa taught me that the soul of a person with Alzheimer's disease still sings and paints and dances and writes and portrays itself to all who truly perceive. There remains a story to "tell," though the affliction of cognitive impairment may alter the voice, making it unrecognizable to even the speaker at times. But I am convinced there is no greater privilege in this world than to help another person find and express his/her true voice, and no greater crime than to silence it.

We all have richly-woven life stories. Like a memory quilt, these stories are meant to be shared and felt. They can bring comfort, along with a blood stain or two. But they must not be left in the cedar chest. Such treasure is too fine for rot and moth. We need the warmth of home found in their weave. And all quilt makers need their work to be loved and valued.

It took very little time during my visit to the Michigan Alzheimer's Disease Center and Cognitive Disorders Clinics in 2012 to realize how special the place, and its directors, staff, patients, and care givers are. There is such an atmosphere of affirmation and validation there; a focus on living life as richly as possible in every moment we are given. And the Center is determined to provide all the tools and support needed to make life quality as good as it can be. I actually felt a sense of personal wellness just being there and interacting with those fine people.

And here, showcased on these pages, true to form, they have taken things soaring to another level altogether. Contained herein are memories, emotions, quilts and paintings, songs and stories, lilting dance and weary plodding, blacks and whites, darks and lights, the rain and sun of life in this world. All expressed through the realities of affliction, unfiltered, unframed, and untethered.

And on each page, in each emotive line, the light of personhood illuminates the dark of human affliction, revealing a multi-faceted diamond of the self. The treasure of each life, to be seen, touched, known.

And when we all reach in to cherish the find, we join hands with the rest of humanity. And that is the only way we win.

So open the chest, wrap up in some quilts, and behold the hidden treasures of life and memory contained herein. As you do, remember the lives, remember the stories, pass them down to the young ones. In doing so we honor our elders, validate ourselves, and inspire our children.

Daniel C. Potts, M.D.

Founder and President, Cognitive Dynamics Foundation
www.cognitivedynamics.org

ACKNOWLEDGMENTS

We are very grateful to the Michigan Alzheimer's Disease Center for financially supporting this publication. The advice and editorial assistance we received from Jasna Markovac, Senior Advisor of Publishing and Related Business Development at the University of Michigan Medical School, was invaluable. We appreciate Nancy North's skillful contributions as copyeditor and Terri Geitgey's assistance and support throughout the publication process. Leigh Sugar and Abby Sugar provided helpful instructions for starting this project. Lynette Girbach kept us organized and on track, and we thank her for her diligence. Some of our authors received assistance from several very special individuals who work with them regularly and who provided encouragement and writing coaching. We acknowledge Kathi Tobey and Elaine Reed for their devoted assistance.

Some of the creative contributions to this collection were the result of interviews completed during an elective narrative medicine class by second-year University of Michigan medical students with members of the U-M Geriatrics Center's Silver Club Programs. We want to acknowledge both students and Club members for the invaluable experience they provided for each other. We thank each artist and interviewee for providing permission for us to publish these works. Names and some personal details have been altered by the authors to maintain privacy and allow for creative interpretation.

Members of the Silver Club and Elderberry Club Programs provided the artwork included in this collection. Students of the U-M School of Art and Design, working with Professor Anne Mondro, provided artistic support.

We thank each and every author and artist for contributing to this community effort. And we thank you, the reader, for your interest.

Perspectives of those who live with memory loss

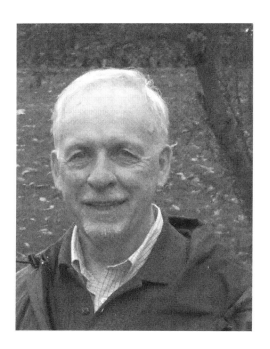

Ken Saulter was born and raised in Cleveland, Ohio. He received his PhD in Economics from the University of California, Santa Barbara in 1976. He spent his professional career working largely with government and nonprofit research organizations. In his spare time, Ken ran 14 marathons. He is married to Diane Saulter and together they raised two, now married, sons.

GOOD FORTUNE

Ken Saulter

I've had a lot of good fortune in my life. I was able to survive an abusive father, get through high school and college on my own, have a satisfying career, have a terrific family with my wife and two sons, and mostly excellent health over 60 years.

When I think about my professional good fortune four events stand out, and, in particular four phone calls that offered opportunities that shaped my career and literally transformed my life.

The first was from my boss in Cleveland asking if I would be interested in leaving a Johnson & Johnson sales territory in Flint, Michigan, for a territory in Sacramento covering all of Northern California.

The second call was from the University of California, Santa Barbara, when the Chairman of the Economics Department asked if I would commit to entering the UCSB Graduate PhD Economics program with a three-year teacher's assistant stipend.

The third call was from my dissertation advisor. Would I be interested in spending a year in Washington, DC on a Ford Foundation Energy Policy Project working as a staff economist?

And lastly, there was the call from a State Department official asking if I would I be interested in accepting a senior staff position with the United Nations Geneva office of the Economic Commission for Europe.

These four opportunities cover the period 1963 to 1976, a little over 10 years, and influenced the rest of my professional life and fulfilled a life-long dream to live abroad.

My professional life came to an end when I was given what many people would consider the worst possible news. But what might have been the end of my good fortune, has turned out to be a new set of learning opportunities.

The bad news was not delivered over the phone. It was delivered in person and ineptly by a doctor, a neurologist, in his office. The doctor told us -- in a rather cold way, sitting across a long office room, and talking over his

3

right shoulder -- that I had Alzheimer's disease and he was sorry to be the one to tell me. My wife, Diane, asked some questions and received discouraging answers. In particular the doctor said that support groups are usually not helpful. We walked out of the neurologist's office without information, without direction, and without hope.

This was unacceptable. It felt like having a verdict of terminal cancer in the 1950s.

We began researching the Ann Arbor area for medical information and family support. And found an abundance of resources via the University of Michigan and the local chapter of the Alzheimer's Association.

Within the next months we had joined the "Coffeehouse" support group at the U-M for individuals with Mild Cognitive Impairment (MCI), joined a research project investigating long-term memory decline, donated my brain to science, AND joined a group in the neighborhood to do a white water rafting adventure down the Grand Canyon Colorado River.

As soon as I could, I began meeting with the Coffeehouse group and became aware of the available medical and care-giving resources and how large the Alzheimer's community was. We definitely were not alone! The fears that I had about my life narrowing and fading away soon were dispelled, at least for now.

We soon realized that telling me I had Alzheimer's was premature, and that living with Mild Cognitive Impairment can be a time full of opportunity and personal growth.

As a member of the Coffeehouse group I've had opportunities to learn about the brain from leading researchers in the field. I've learned both about brain diseases and ways to keep the brain as healthy as possible. I've had opportunities to contribute feedback to health care professionals from the point of view of seniors with cognitive issues and opportunities to speak at conferences for health care professionals.

Coffeehouse is a unique opportunity to learn about the neurology field and how it responds to our questions and concerns. Experts who attended our meetings tried to answer our questions and were, in effect, validating our roles as patient advocates, not solely medical health-care patients.
The participants in the MCI group develop close and caring
relationships, and as a senior member of the group I've had a lot of satisfaction learning for myself and helping others to learn.

Life is still stimulating because of the kinds of opportunities that appear from day to day and week to week. My wife amazes me with her determination to help me find activities and connections that actually add to my life rather than detract from it in spite of my physical and cognitive limitations. (Two years after that premature Alzheimer's disease diagnosis I was diagnosed with Parkinson's.)

In addition to my Coffeehouse experiences, I've enjoyed the support and encouragement that comes from members of an Osher Lifelong Learning Institute memoir writing group. Over the last three years I've written about my life and listened to the writing of others that has helped me express myself and feel satisfaction that I'm not just a marginal member of my community. Participating in the writing group is difficult at times, but nevertheless it's an opportunity to express myself as long as I can.

My early experiences in my teen years in particular had to do with sports; sports were a valuable learning tool. Now, in my late years, writing, particularly writing and listening to fellow members' writing, has been the principal means to learning of my inner life.

I am grateful for the opportunities I've had to be a mentor to others with MCI as I participate in Coffeehouse. I believe more understanding of these diseases can help alleviate the anxiety we experience as we face the future. We are bringing the "Muhammad Ali and Michael J. Fox learning and caring" to our own community.

BETWEEN US

Ken Saulter

Losing my memory,
Losing my memory to a terminal disease,
Is getting to be a problem.

Like when I'm in a group
And people talk to me and then,
Suddenly, I fall silent,
While my brain, and my heart, skip a beat.

We know it's not a so-called senior moment.
Eyes divert to shoe laces or thereabouts,
Anywhere else but the ceiling.
The moment becomes one of palpable discomfort.

So here I am, a fraction of a man,
A clown without make-up or costume,
Waiting giant seconds to recover.

I'm told I will not remember these bricks of separation
In the wall that is, regrettably, being built between us.

I worry a lot about little things, like forgetting
My locker combination, after 20+ years of use.
--- Or forgetting large things, like the names of my sons,
--- Or maybe someday, the address where I live,
--- Or, luckily, maybe not.

But, against our wills,
The wall keeps getting higher and higher.

Still, I'll keep on living, accepting losses and
Focusing on what I've got -- and you.

Meanwhile I'll keep trying to lower the wall between us,
--- Or slow it down,
--- Or build a gate,
--- Or do something.

Ken Saulter writes: "These ideas were inspired by what I learned at the 2009 Edna Gates Conference. This poem explores the idea of dementia as the wearing of an internal mask worn every day. It also recognizes the important role that caregivers serve by supporting and encouraging personal expression among those who have to deal with the burden of the mask and the struggle to keep one's identity."

MY MASK AND I

Ken Saulter

I look out through my mask occasionally,
To see who is there or if I have to speak. Can you see me?

Too bad my voice is so broken, but my mask and I
Know who I am. Can you hear me?

I've lost a lot of memories, but plenty remain.
My mask and I stand stoically as memories shift in and out.
Do you know who I am?

The world is smaller with a heavy mask on, and where is my smile?

Where is the touch of my hand? Will I always feel lonely?
My body and mind grow stiff. My mask and I know why.
Maybe I'll turn to stone someday. Will I learn anything, anymore?

I look out through my mask, occasionally,
To see who is there or if I have to speak.
My voice keeps getting smaller. Can you hear me?

And my body becomes less and less.
Can you touch my hand? Must I take that pill?

And then, suddenly, someone different looks at me
And hears me and smiles at me and I see things in a new way.

And I become more, rather than less.
And my mask melts day after day and
People look at me directly and see me as I am.
And there's no more "through a mask" living.
The table has turned as has the burden of the mask.

... Do you see the bright colors I've chosen for my canvas?

... Isn't my voice strong?

... Yes, and I see that you are listening to me now!

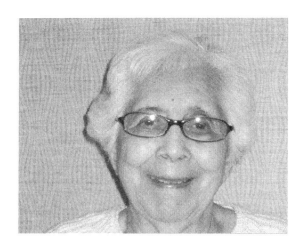

Josephine Moreno was born in Dallas, Texas in 1923. She came to Michigan, to a new way of life awaiting her and her family. As she describes it, "We lived in the country with no electricity, no gas for cooking and heating, and no running water. I met my husband, Daniel, in Mt. Pleasant, Michigan. We were the proud parents of four children. At present, I am a widow and very content living in an assisted living community near Lake Michigan."

HOW I LEARNED TO SPEAK ENGLISH – AN ELEMENTARY SCHOOL MEMORY

Josephine Moreno

I grew up speaking Spanish. It was not until I went to Michigan that I recall hearing English spoken for the first time. Our family always spoke Spanish in our home. This is what I remember.

It was April 1928 when our family left Dallas, Texas, for Michigan. There were five children in our family and I was the youngest, only being four years old. So, the few oldest ones were sad about the move to Michigan. Dallas was a large city. There they had attended school and there were things they were involved with in junior high. I, being the youngest, only knew that school days were ahead for me, and I was too young to think about this.

Things I recall on the trip: There were two buses traveling together with people hoping to find work in Michigan. They were told there was work in Michigan. We did not stop at restaurants. We were given food that the bus company was providing. They served sardines often. And to this day, I don't care for them.

How many days it took to travel, I don't recall. We crossed the Mississippi River on a ferry on a cold afternoon. Somewhere on the road there was an accident on one of the buses, and people were injured. There was a delay on the trip. We finally arrived in Michigan. It was an April spring day. Our family was taken to the William Bradley farm near Prattville, Michigan. It was a small village. We were given a tenant house on the farm to begin our home life in Michigan. This was where I heard the English language in conversation for the first time. Of course I didn't know what they were saying, it was "foreign" to me!

One day Mrs. Bradley came to ask permission if I could come to her house for lunch. Their granddaughter, Roberta, was coming there to visit. So my sister took me there. We were greeted by Mrs. Bradley, and she said, "Josephine can have anything on the table she wishes to eat, but must say it in English." So, then she pointed to each dish a few times saying in English what the food was. And we sat at the table.

The only thing I could remember to say was potato. I said something like this, "Pasa de potato por favor!" That meant, "Pass the potato please!" My first word in English was potato.

Mrs. Bradley gave me anything else I wanted. I was nervous and shaky. My sister went with me. I had never been in an English-speaking house. After the meal, Roberta and I had a nice time becoming acquainted and getting to know one another. I couldn't speak English and she couldn't speak Spanish, but that was not any problem. We had a good time. Kids can get along with no problem.

We lived there until fall. My father asked if we could please move to where there was a school so my sister and brother could attend. They moved us to Waldron, Michigan. We lived there a short while and then they moved us to Metamora, Ohio. That was 1929 and I was old enough to attend first grade.

My sister and brother were in the eighth and ninth grades. They took me to the lower level to start grade school. I was introduced to Miss Zimmerman, the first grade teacher. They spoke to her in English, which I did not understand. Then they went to their class room and left me with the rest of the first grade class.

She started the day by singing, "Jesus Wants Me for a Sunbeam." When I heard that tune, I recognized the tune. I softly sang the words in Spanish while they sang in English. We also sang at noon, for lunch time, and at the end of the school day before dismissal. I knew something was about to happen whenever we sang.

Then she taught me to raise my finger to go for a drink or to the bathroom. She would use a lot of gesturing to help me. So my days of learning began. After the morning song, it was game time. I would watch all the others as they played. They played a game that was a skipping game. The boy would come and bow to the girl, and they would skip to the music. I didn't understand the skipping game. I went home and told my mother that a little boy asked me to play a skipping game. My sister overheard me talking to my mother. She said, "The boy who asked you to skip is named Roy, and his sister is in his class." Roy's sister was in my sister's class. She told Roy to, "Be kind to Josephine!"

Miss Zimmerman wanted me to feel comfortable. On the first day, she gave me many flash cards with pictures and words in English on them. Later, I was learning my ABCs and how to read. I listened and followed along as best I could. I took a book home to read. My sister helped me learn to read. I learned my reading lesson by heart. I still know it today. It goes like this,

Alice said, "Come cat, come to dinner."

And the cat said, "No. We will find our dinner."

That came from the Edson Reader, a blue book. Miss Zimmerman was not fooled. She knew it from memory. But the lessons became easier and easier as I learned more and more of the English language. When you are little and eager to learn, it stays with you. Learning numbers and counting came next. Then we learned to write our name in cursive. That was a lot to learn in nine months of first grade. This is especially true for someone who didn't speak English at the beginning of the year. I learned English because the students spoke to me in English. They were helpful in teaching correct pronunciation. I passed the first grade!

Miss Brian was my second grade teacher and we read stories and did arithmetic. I can't say if I spoke English fluently, but I certainly understood it in second grade. I was always interested in learning something new. I was learning more difficult words and how they were pronounced correctly. I learned the pledge of allegiance in second grade.

In third grade I had Mrs. Hackett. She taught more difficult reading lessons. We started using the library to get books. The librarian would help me choose a book. I remember reading about Hansel and Gretel. There was a play put on by the school at the Methodist Church auditorium. They presented the play Hansel and Gretel, and I was one of the children in the play.

The reading books became harder in third grade. We had an orange-colored school book called, "A Journey to Healthland." It was all about cleanliness. It taught us everything about taking care of your body from brushing your teeth to combing your hair. It was my favorite book and I kept it for a long time.

As I recall these memories, others are starting to flood my brain. I remember stories about Billy Goat Gruff, Jack and the Beanstalk, and Little Red Riding Hood. I am really thankful for my first teachers and how they taught me to speak English. Now, if I could only remember what I had for breakfast.

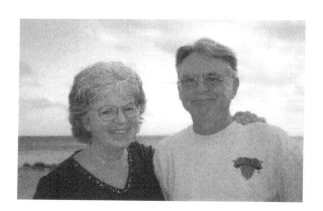

Phil and Pam have been married for 47 years. They met at Swarthmore College, raised three wonderful daughters, and are active with Friends (Quaker) organizations. They are both retired—Phil from Ford, Pam from counseling practice and parenting education in order to spend more time painting. They feel grateful for family, friends, and many blessings.

WANDERING TOGETHER

Pam and Phil Hoffer

My husband and I have decided to share a bit about an unwanted journey, which began in 2008, that we find ourselves on. We hope that sharing our attempts to navigate this unknown territory will be useful, perhaps first to us and our family, but maybe to others as well.

Conversation
(Journal Entries - January, 2011)

Do you remember anything about that first appointment and the first memory testing?

No, I don't. [long silence] I kinda remember not being able to remember a sequence of numbers and I kind of dismiss that as 'why would I want to remember random numbers anyway,' but that is probably just a defense mechanism. But whatever it was, that was frustrating. I still feel real gratitude for you getting me into the doctor and the research studies. I'm sure I'm better off for doing that and getting on a program to exercise more and get the medicine early to maybe ameliorate all this, even if I can't do anything about the genes I inherited.

Can I jump in here to describe that first appointment? It was REALLY an eye opener for me. THANK GOODNESS for the kindness of the doctor. I was right there with you while the mini-cognitive test was administered. If I had not witnessed that little test and ONLY been given the results it would NOT have had anywhere NEAR the useful and important impact that it did. It was "world shifting" for me.

It wasn't the numbers that gave you trouble, honey. You aced all that part. You were given five nouns to remember, told you could rehearse them, which you did, told you would be asked to repeat them a few minutes later. Then the doctor chatted with you a bit and in a few minutes asked you to recall the five nouns. I knew you had paid attention, saw you rehearse them with clear intention to remember them, and then, you could not recall ONE. Nor could you experience remembering them when offered choices – is it a church, a hospital or a school? You thought really hard, and said to each set of choices, "I don't know, but if I had to guess, I would say...." And then you picked the right noun! But you did NOT have the Aha! recognition of the right word. That just blew me away. And two things happened right away: First, it made me totally and scarily aware that a real

15

problem was going on. And second, and really importantly, a few years of anger I had felt toward you for forgetting our conversations and decisions—all that anger just melted and dropped totally away.

We have talked a lot about why we might want to share openly, and I can wax on and on about reasons, but what is your thinking?

Oh! My thinking is because I might get some beneficial helpful hints that might come back to me if I am open and there is no reason not to admit to a deteriorated memory. If I were in junior high or something, it would be a real stigma not having a memory. I know it is not my fault; there is probably a genetic component.

I am ready to spend more time making sure that we get a lot of time in with good friends and family, in whatever context, working or walking or playing. And my own feeling is that whatever stigma does attach to Alzheimer's, being open about our situation allows for some of that stigma to be blown out of the water. This early stage we are in has not disturbed our daily lives very much and need not be so terribly frightening. And if we are transparent about it, maybe others can be a little less frightened and get themselves checked out early if they are experiencing significant changes. I am just so grateful to have information early enough that I have been able to take on some major new roles with your help and not wait until that help was not available from you.

At some point, if I really deteriorate, I might say something embarrassing, and that might have an effect on our friendships. I just don't know what my physical or social condition is going to be in the future. But if it gets bad, I don't believe I will be seen as contagious. And if I start acting inappropriately, I can cut back on my social interactions.

Well, if there are those that are worried about contagion, we can let those friendships shake out now and make room to deepen ones that hold and even make room for new ones. Sometimes I get "down" and feel like our lives have begun to shrink.

What do you mean? We are still making room for new experiences, like deciding to go more often to Live at the Metropolitan Opera programs when they come to [the movie theater].

True! And that's been delightful.

What Slips Away
(Journal Entry - March 15th, 2011)

Phil is now in his second year on medication and we expect Alzheimer's is the culprit, even though the diagnosis is Mild Cognitive Impairment. The progression is slow-ish. He is still a very warm, witty presence in social situations because he can be in the moment. BUT, it really is changing. And as that has happened, bits of my identity feel as though they are slipping away.

Recently I had a chance to talk with a lovely woman I was introduced to through a friend. This woman's husband had died of Alzheimer's and all throughout their journey, there was another woman with the same experience behind her who had been her mentor. It was such a help to her that she decided after her husband died to do the same mentoring for someone else. When we met, I told her about how quickly I had been coming to tears (I have always been really leaky that way). I was feeling like it was grieving and thought I would get through it. Her really helpful comment was, "Well, you are going to be grieving for a long, long time with many losses ahead and you don't need to wait until that is done. It won't be for a long time. So you don't have to wait."

After that conversation, I went to the pharmacist, asked him what he noted about the various antidepressants, and got information about prices and dosage. Then I talked with my primary care doctor about trying the lowest possible dose of something just to give me a BOWL to carry my feelings in, instead of carrying them in what has felt like a PLATE, with spillage just too easy. Years ago, before my father died, he had asked me to read a message at his memorial service that he wrote to his friends. It was quite beautiful, and as leaky as I am I knew I would choke up and cry and make a mess of it, making my tears what was noticed instead of his words. I asked my doctor for a pill that would allow me to get through this task without breaking down. What she gave me worked like a charm and allowed me to read his lovely message adequately. So I knew about the "Bowl" phenomenon. My wonderful doctor knew what I needed, and within two days I felt the difference. I woke the second day with a slight headache (most unusual) and thought, "Aha, the medicine at work!" And over the last few days, which have contained a number of conversations in which I would have gotten all teary, I simply HAVEN'T.

It is clear that there are unexpected gifts as well as losses in this process. In addition to the personal challenge and reward of growing up further, the process of memory loss in these stages clarifies the importance of finding joy in the present moments. Phil has always been able to find joy easily, and that remains his great talent, undiminished by the process so far, and he remains my teacher in this respect.

Sharing with Our Congregation: Ann Arbor Friends Meeting – April 2011

Dear Friends,

Pam and I have been considering for some time an idea to write a letter together for the newsletter briefly summarizing our current life and medical challenge revolving around my diagnosis of memory loss. We do this in the spirit of openness because we know that important help has already come to us by being open and having shared what is going on with a number of friends. Also because we would want to encourage others to confront any similar difficulties as early as possible. I am lucky to have gotten medical care EARLY, when it is likely to be of most help. We know that our demographic group is likely to encounter problems of memory and cognitive decline, so we definitely don't feel alone.

Our lives have not changed in many respects, but early diagnosis has allowed me to turn over to Pam tasks that I used to do, and I am still able to help her in that transition. We feel a lot of love and support from friends and are happy to share with others anything we learn along the way that might be useful to others. Feel free to talk to us about all this. There is a phrase we have encountered – "The Grace of Diminishment" – that seems to be helpful to keep in mind.

With love and trust,
Phil

SWEETHEART

Pam Hoffer

"Where does all this rain come from?" you ask,
"Is it coming out of the clouds?"
The question is stunning
Your beginner's mind,
Regained innocence,
Preserved curiosity
And your sweet acceptance of not knowing,
Though you are seventy-two and a Harvard grad.

This journey backward, or so it would seem,
Yet stumbles toward enlightenment.
How strange to habitate the present moment
without the monk's lifetime of discipline.

And do I ask such questions or even detect
All that I ignore not knowing, missing out on that beginner mind,
Steering our course by habit and invention.

We rely on each other, going this distance.
I remember a couple I worked with years ago
fragile in their old age and each with Parkinson's
and its festinating gait.
One tended to fall backward, the other forward.
And they could proceed just fine together
When aligned just right.

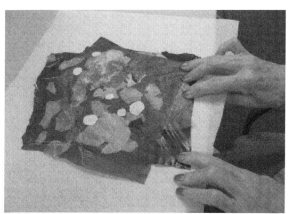

Reprinted with permission from Club Member, Silver Club Programs, U-M Geriatrics Center

The Elderberry Club (Elder, barely) was originally formed in September 2011 as one of the University of Michigan Geriatrics Center's Silver Club Programs. This group of younger women has been meeting weekly to support, educate and share their experiences of living with early onset memory loss. They are a group of vibrant women who are interested in a social gathering for cultural enrichment, expression and creativity.

ELDERBERRY CLUB

Kathi Tobey, Elaine Reed, Members of the Elderberry Club

We are women,
gathered in kindness,
living well and
living with memory loss.

We are creative,
supportive, connected
caring, sharing, exploring,
fun-loving, courageous and

Full of Hope....

EVERMORE

Kathi Tobey, Elaine Reed, Members of the Elderberry Club

Evermore…
Learning and Loving
Determined
Endeavoring to excel
Respecting ourselves

Beautiful women inside and out
Abiding hope
Resilient
Ever thankful
Living out our dreams
Young in life!

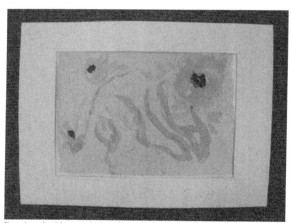

Reprinted with permission from Club Member, Silver Club Programs, U-M Geriatrics Center

The Wisdom Keepers is one of several groups within the University of Michigan Geriatrics Center's Silver Club Programs. Wisdom Keepers is a talented group of multi-aged men & women who are living well with memory loss. They meet weekly for lively reminiscence and friendship, and they are interested in topical discussions, creative projects, outings and social enrichment.

WISDOM KEEPER

Kathi Tobey, Elaine Reed, Members of the Wisdom Keepers Group

Wisdom we impart to others:
Learn from and enjoy each other
Make the most of your time
Decide what really matters to you
Keep in touch with your friends

Who we are:
We are good listeners and interested in learning new things
We're happy people and love to laugh
The young people in our families are our pride and joy
We are open to new ideas and are willing to share
We enjoy life!

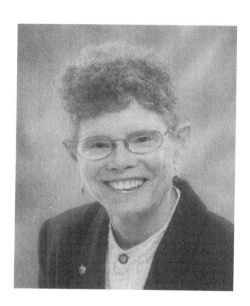

Gretchen L. Smith has worked in creative writing and photography for both profit and non-profit organizations over her 40-year career. More than 14 years of that time were spent in non-profit health care. She has a bachelor's degree from Ball State University, is a Distinguished Toastmaster and a graduate of the National Speakers' Association-Michigan Pro-Track Program. To keep her mind active, she has started her own public speaking and writing business – Outside the Lines Communications, LLC.

TICK, TOCK

Gretchen Smith

Tick, tick, tick, tick...blank computer screen: I know the word I want to use. I can see it, but my hands won't let me tap the keys to put it on paper. I stare at the screen fiercely, willing my brain to cough up that word. A half-hour passes. Use a word that's acceptable, close to what I want to say, and maybe the real word will come to me.

I was given a diagnosis with early stage Alzheimer's in December 2008. Nice Christmas present! The doctor asked me several questions after I told him about my trouble with word capture. He gave me some prescriptions and sent me to see a neuropsychologist.

Since that day, I've had three neuropsychological exams and blood work showing I carry the protein that codes for the Apo4 gene associated with Alzheimer's disease. In a pre-screen for a clinical trial I was informed I do not have early-stage Alzheimer's, but Mild Cognitive Impairment.

Most people think it's great I have just Mild Cognitive Impairment. I get a lot of, "Oh, it's part of the aging process. I forget things all the time." I've been asked: "How do you know it's Mild Cognitive Impairment and not just aging?"

My answer is two-fold: First, there was a sentinel moment when I realized that some insidious synapse had derailed my ability to recall descriptive words. Second, Elizabeth Kubler-Ross beautifully outlines the five stages of loss or grief. I am still in Big Denial, Anger and Bargaining after five years.

Let me take you inside the world of someone with Mild Cognitive Impairment whose clock is ticking.

As I began to put my thoughts down, I started with a long narrative history. I became very frustrated because this took me six hours – something that ordinarily I would have written in a half hour. And when I looked at it, my first thought was, "This is crap and says nothing about my inner world."

Every day I struggle with taking the steps needed to jump-start my professional speaking and writing business I've been working on for two years. I know I have to learn social media, but it's like a foreign language to me. I know I need to do this to get myself known. But change is hard, especially when you're afraid you're going to fail.

I make lists everyday – sometimes multiple lists – just to keep myself on task. Everything I must do goes in my calendar and on my phone. I just have to figure out how to set up alerts on my phone. Technology should be easy – it's a big mobile mountain I'm still climbing. I have to re-read everything I write multiple times because I will often put down a very different word than the one I meant – and spell-check will not catch that. I'm not typing a hundred words a minute. I know what I want to say, but my mind keeps putting in words different than what I think I've written.

I used to be able to multi-task and keep 10 projects in mind – what had been done and what yet needed to be done. Now I have file folders for every project. And every scrap of information or communications gets printed out and put in the folder. I can no longer rely on finding the right information in my email or even in my computer file folders. I forget where I put things.

I've lost a cell phone and several presents because I can't recall where I stashed them. Every cord to anything is labeled. I've finally set up a list of passwords because I can't remember which password I've used for which account.

My mind wanders during the day, and it requires every ounce of energy to pull my mind back to a task and keep going. I used to be able to get up early in the morning and go until late at night. Now, it's a struggle to be up before 7 a.m. and stay awake beyond 10 p.m.

I used to be able to rip off addresses and phone numbers without thinking. If it's not in my contact book, you won't be hearing from me. I am a voracious reader, and yet I'm unlikely to be able to tell you the plot of a book I've just read. I had to give up on "Life of Pi" because I was lost on page 10. I've read all the classics and never had any trouble following those plot lines, so fiction is dubious for me. If the plot is too complicated, I just get lost.

I've always valued that my word is a pledge. Now, I'm faced with having to choose just how much volunteer energy I can give. It's easy with Mild Cognitive Impairment to bury yourself in volunteer tasks, and abandon what's most important. For me, it's starting a business that encourages individuals to stretch their intention span and to pay things forward. I don't know how many days, months or years I have before I will lose the cognitive abilities I still have. So, I'm pulling back from volunteering because I don't have the time to let myself dawdle in tasks that require constant contact and follow-up.

I've always hated meetings, but I finally left a service club because their meetings were running two and one-half hours, decisions were being delayed until more information was gathered. I'm at a point now that any meeting, even a conference call, better be done in an hour, and there better be some action steps as a result. I'm losing the patience I once had for long deliberations. I think of myself as a calm, mindful and meditative person. Now, I encounter this impatient person who is often angry (mostly at myself) and anxious most of the time.

Most people – even those who know me fairly well – think there's nothing wrong with me. They see the high-achieving person they've known. That's because they're not inside my brain. I can be in conversation and if someone interrupts, and the conversation starts again, I'm probably lost because my train of thought has been interrupted.

I can't attend functions where there are more than 20 people around with whom I have to converse. There's just too much remembering who I have been introduced to and what has been said, and yet my goal is to lead workshops and seminars where there are hopefully more than 20 people attending. That's going to require energy, a high attention focus, a notebook, and participants interacting with me. And I will leave feeling drained.

Let me leave you with a few final thoughts. I can't imagine not knowing who I am, or who is with me, or not having something to do. The end result of dementia or Alzheimer's is a body whose organs are functioning, but the mind has left on permanent vacation. I am struggling with myself on this issue. I know what the theological perspective is. I've seen how devastating it is to caregivers to devote precious years to assisting loved ones who don't have a clue about who they are or their daily life. This is frightening to someone whose life has centered around using her mind. Yet there it is….tick, tock, tick, tock.

Leslie Rzeznik is a University of Michigan BA candidate in English, sub-concentration in Creative Writing: Poetry. She was the winner of the Undergraduate Academy of American Poets Award at Michigan for Fall 2012. She suffered a traumatic brain injury six years ago and is working on a poetic series based on her recovery. Some of the poems are featured in this anthology. Ms. Rzeznik's work has previously been published in translation in Lithuania; this is her first publication in English.

STALL

Leslie Rzeznik

She pitches forward

The moment
stalls like a plane at two
thousand feet
that lands safely but breaks
the pilot's neck as it flips
in a rut on the ground

Soon she'll be picking words
from between carpet tufts
that stink with the soles
of two thousand feet

BRAIN KISSES BONE SO HARD IT FORGETS WHAT IT IS

Leslie Rzeznik

What does it mean to mistake
a violet for a jackhammer?

Thought is a heavy vaulted door
that shuts when a dust mote lands
just so then right in the middle of my....

I can't stand to listen to myself but can't stop
talking can't stand to listen to myself.

Others' words read clear and true, but my own
trip and shudder off my tongue, thick and dumb.

My shoulder tics in time with every fractured syllable.

Like an owl casing prey,
each swallow or turn of the head spins
my voice from right to wrong.

The unending hisssssss.

I wish I could unhinge my jaw.

APPROACHING JOY

Leslie Rzeznik

"She's been mute for 10 years," they said.

Joy's fingertips linger as she walks. They pantomime Bach or Mozart or perhaps even "Muskrat Love." In those moments when they are perfectly still, I catch an essence of baby kisses or clean-running river water over her outstretched palm, running past the fetal lifemarks of hopes and loves, slipping under the wedding ring (not hers) and evaporating before it hits dimensional reality.

Her spirit protected by neglect and isolation, it's more free than yours or mine, embalmed as ours have been by society's engenderment and cultural morés and spirit-numbing sameness. Joy's eyes bore into your face, staring deep past your molars as you speak, but parking on your pupils during the in-between breaths, as if she'll be able to catch a glimpse of an as-yet-undeveloped photograph if she cannot blink in the split seconds while the aperture flashes.

You wonder if she understands, but find it difficult to be anything but forthcoming under her gaze. She nods and smiles politely in all the right places. Anyone observing the conversation from afar might think she's a particularly engaged companion, that your story is so compelling that she wouldn't think to interrupt. You wonder if she thinks. And if she does, what she thinks.

You get the feeling she knows you. That if she could just talk, she could tell you stories about yourself. Like how you got that scar under your chin that you kept forgetting to ask your mother about before she died. Or that maybe you used to waltz or jitterbug together that summer when you were 17 and developed a sudden but short-lived case of sleepwalking. You dreamt of dancing shadows, but was it Joy?

Joy hasn't spoken, but she laughs. No titters or coy giggles for Joy. Her laugh is befitting of her name. It's deep and swallows anyone within earshot. You're either embarrassed or delighted by her laugh. If you don't laugh with her, sometimes it transmutes into a strange uncontrolled caterwaul, and you're afraid she's going to pee her pants or suffocate herself, and wonder just what you'll do then if you're out in public.

Joy rarely laughs at inappropriate moments. She never laughs at anyone, unless they're already laughing at themselves. Occasionally she turns what could be a decidedly embarrassing moment into an amusing anecdote – just with her laughter. It's sometimes easy to forget she's not quite there with you.

So where is she and how did she get there and will she ever be coming back?

She loves fabric stores. Loves to run those kinetic fingers over linens and wools and printed cottons. She loves the smell of raw silk and screws her face up at polyester. Burlap makes her laugh and flop her hands from the ends of her wrists. She can stand for an hour testing the hand of a silk charmeuse, watching it flow over her fingers like a liquid sand sculpture, again and again. Perhaps she had been a seamstress.

Music makes her seem less otherworldly. Sometimes I'll take her to a nightclub just because she enjoys it so much. She moves and sways like she once had a dancer's body, but mis- or under-use and age have caged her. I can see the men watching her with desire and the women with envy. But never jealousy. She has this gift of being completely engaging from a distance. Strangers are surprised, sometimes offended at first when her lips part only to show her perfect teeth in a perfect smile. Some have the disrespect to ask me pointblank what's wrong with her, as if she were not sitting right next to us.

That's the only time I ever see her agitated, and seems to be one of the few indicators that she not only understands, but can be hurt, by someone's thoughtlessness. I've never seen her cry. She just gets very quiet. Her movement stops. Like a small sleepy child, she rubs her eyes and I know it's time for us to leave.

Back in her room, if it's been a good night, she'll turn on the radio and twirl and dip while she brushes her teeth. She'll let me brush her hair and sometimes French braid it, even though I know it will come undone by the morning. If she's had her feelings hurt, she'll go right to sleep without even changing her clothes. If she were little enough or I were strong enough, I think she'd doze off in the car and let me carry her sleep-grogged form directly to bed, sour breath and all.

Before I leave, I make sure she's tucked in tight, but not too tight, kiss her forehead, and promise her I'll be back same time next week. If the day ever comes when she's able or decides to participate in conversation again, I wonder if I'll miss her silence.

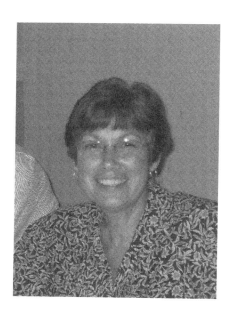

Myriam Torres holds a Masters of Statistics and worked more than 25 years as a research associate at the Institute of Social Research at the University of Michigan, where she received several honors. She recently retired due to developing Alzheimer's. Myriam also served as a lay Christian pastoral worker and founding member of Bethany Association, an ecumenical group of women living single for the Lord. She told her story with a little help from her friends.

WHEN YOUR WORST FEAR BECOMES REALITY

Myriam Torres

My first big clue that something was very wrong came in February 2009. I was on a Christian mission trip to Costa Rica, meeting with a small group of women. Suddenly I couldn't understand a word they were saying. I didn't let on, but I was totally at a loss. All I could do was make a comment every now and then and hope it was all right. I got some puzzled looks, but somehow I made it through the next hour. Afterwards, I reverted to normal.

Things weren't normal, though, when I got back home. I cried all the time without knowing why. In my job as a high-level statistician, I found myself struggling to analyze data and needing to delegate my work to other analysts. "Could be menopause," a friend suggested. I was fifty-six and had already gone through that stage, so it didn't seem likely. "Stress," thought someone else. I took a month off from work, but things only got worse.

A nurse practitioner urged me to see a doctor, and so began two years of medical tests. Early on, after a psychological test revealed "significant" mental impairments, one specialist noted, "probably Alzheimer's disease." If I ever read his comment, I dismissed it right away.

That diagnosis wasn't confirmed until May 2011. By that time, because of my increasing confusion and forgetfulness, I had left the job I loved. And I was wrestling with God in a very serious way.

But I'm Your Bride!

For most of my adult life, I've lived "single for the Lord" as part of an ecumenical group of women who have chosen not to marry in order to dedicate ourselves to a life of prayer and Christian service. And so, though we work at various professions and don't take religious vows, I see myself as a bride of Christ, deeply loved and deeply in love with Jesus.

Every day before work, I used to get up to spend an hour with him. I loved it. I'd praise and worship God singing, reading Scripture, reflecting, and writing down things that struck me. But as I felt myself declining, I became very angry with the Lord. "Is this the way you treat your bride?" I'd ask him. But he was silent.

Deep down, I knew that if I refused to choose "your way, not mine," I was the one who was going to be the loser. Still, for nearly two years I fought and struggled. I denied what was happening, tried to cover up, refused to discuss it. With all my heart I wanted to believe that my problem was sleep deprivation, stress, or even depression – anything but Alzheimer's.

This wrestling went on and on, but at least I kept talking to the Lord. Then one day, during my prayer time, he gave me an unexpected grace. I suddenly realized that I could really trust him with my future. "I accept this," I told Jesus very simply. The peace I felt got me through the final medical consultation, which left no doubt that I have progressive dementia: Alzheimer's disease, according to one last test.

Sherry, a close friend who is also single for the Lord, was with me as I got the bad news.

"Myriam, you're too quiet," she said, when we were back in the car. "What are you thinking?" "I'm okay. I worked it out with God last night. And I told him it's okay, whatever it is."

Sherry couldn't believe what she was hearing. I could hardly believe it myself. It was pure grace, and so freeing to be able to admit what was happening and to talk about it.

Loved and Loving

After a couple of weeks, I felt like the Lord was asking something more: Thank me. Again I wrestled. Accepting my situation had been hard enough. Did I really have to do this too? It was hard, very hard, but again there came the grace to say yes.

Months later, I realized that I was truly grateful for some of the changes I saw in myself. I'm relating to people differently, in a softer, more loving way. "Thank you, Jesus, for this opportunity." And as I prayed, I sensed a call to go deeper – not just to accept and give thanks, but to embrace the journey with trust in God's love and wisdom. This time my response came easily. I embraced it like a gift from heaven.

This may sound strange, but even as I'm losing my abilities, I'm seeing the "gift" side of what's happening. More and more, all I can do is love and be loved. And I feel so much love from so many people! They're praying for me, telling me what I mean to them, thanking me for ways I've helped them.

And God is still using me to speak words that people need to hear. When women I've counseled over the years call and ask my advice, I usually know what to say. I say it more directly, too, because along with Alzheimer's comes a lessening of inhibitions! I noticed this recently, when a woman in my Zumba exercise class said how worried she was that her husband might have dementia. Not only did I tell her how to get medical help, but right there, with other people listening in, I prayed with her. "I feel so much better now," she said afterwards.

Suffering Servants

Don't get me wrong, though. Embracing this journey isn't the same as embracing the disease. I'm doing all I can to stay fit and slow my decline – speech therapy, exercise, social contacts, a good diet. If God chooses to heal me, I'll be ecstatic. And although I've arrived at a basic peace, there are still struggles and tears. I loved being a statistician, being savvy and capable. Now I can't even count. I can't tell time without a lot of effort. If people talk fast, I can't understand what they say. I have a hard time focusing to pray. It's hard to accept help, too, hard to let go.

An experience I had at the airport last year drove home this sense of loss and helplessness. I was traveling with Sherry, but she went through security just ahead of me, so she couldn't help when I got confused at the guards' directions. I couldn't understand where they wanted me to place my luggage. I didn't know which hand they wanted me to raise. "Don't you know one from the other?" one guard jeered.

I stumbled out of the checkpoint crying. I felt so humiliated. "This is what's coming," I was thinking. "This is the way I'm going to be all the time." Explaining it to Sherry later, I could only say I'd had a taste of what it was like for Jesus, when he was stripped of everything and people were mocking him. I take comfort in the fact that I am being conformed to him. I wrote in my journal, "As time goes on and I lose all I have – the ability to communicate, my memory, being able to do my daily functions--I see that all this is making me more like Jesus, the suffering servant."

St. Ignatius Loyola put it more eloquently in words that I now pray from the heart:

Take, O Lord, and receive all my liberty, my memory, my understanding, and my will, all that I have and possess. You have given all these things to me. To you, Lord, I return them. All are yours. Do with them what you will. Give me only your love and your grace, for that is enough for me.

Reprinted with permission from "The Word Among Us" magazine (January 2013)

IF YOU'RE DEALING WITH MEMORY LOSS

Myriam Torres

Ever since receiving my diagnosis of Alzheimer's disease, I've very actively looked for ways to stay as healthy as possible for as long as possible. I've also become very up front about sharing my findings with anyone who might benefit! Circumstances vary and these may not be for everyone, but here are some of my tips.

Get to a doctor. If you've noticed troubling changes (like the "10 early signs and symptoms" on the Alzheimer's Association website: www.alz.org), but you haven't looked into the cause, go get tested. The sooner you know what you're dealing with, the more time you – and your caregivers – will have to plan and prepare.

Keep moving. Physical exercise helps maintain good blood flow to the brain and has lots of other benefits. I like to go for walks, often with a friend. I've benefited from exercise too. I especially like Qi Gong, a gentle exercise that helps maintain flexibility, balance, and stability and – my number one favorite – Zumba, a Latin dance fitness program. I attend two classes a week and love it!

Eat well. Get those fruits and vegetables, fish, lean meats, and nuts. Enjoy a treat every now and then, but don't overdo it. You'll feel so much better if you have a healthy diet.

Get a pet. Something small that won't be too much work to care for. Mine is a Pomeranian named Zoe. I've never had a dog before, so I'm amazed at what good company she is – fun to play with and alert to anyone at the door. With Zoe around, I never feel alone.

Join a support group. They can be found almost everywhere. Mine is sponsored by the University of Michigan Geriatric Center, and it's been a tremendous help for understanding what is happening to me. There are about 10 men and women in the group, and the social worker who coordinates it is wonderful. We usually share about our daily lives, our questions, struggles, and triumphs. Sometimes we have a speaker – like a pharmacologist who can answer our questions about medications. It's always stimulating and informative. (There are support groups for caregivers, too, by the way.)

Get together with friends. See them as often as you can. Laugh a lot. Have them over, or go out for dinner, a film, a concert (personally, I think music is good for the brain!).

Find a fashion consultant. Maybe it sounds silly, but one of my biggest fears is that I'm going to look ugly. I never know what to put on any more, or what colors go together. When I mentioned this to a good friend one day, she offered to take over. Now she reviews my wardrobe, keeps my closet organized so that I can easily find things that match, and takes me clothes shopping twice a year. She advises me about my hair, too. What a relief!

Ask for help. I've noticed that many people are reluctant to accept help unless they have a way of paying back. But in my background, which is Puerto Rican, we tend to be more direct about expressing our needs. We also expect that family and close friends will help us out even if we can't repay them. I'm not saying that this makes everything easy. Especially in certain areas, I find it very challenging to accept help and relinquish control. But what a blessing to have people who will step in when you need them. So if you have them, ask!

Do crossword and jigsaw puzzles. They're good stimulation. I'm not so good at crosswords any more, but I can still handle a 550-piece jigsaw puzzle and enjoy the challenge.

Prayer helps. Keep talking and listening to God every day. Never neglect him. But find ways of making your prayer time simple and focused. I like going through the daily Mass readings. For a while, I used preloaded mp3 player programs that contain 15 minutes of prayer time for daily use. You could also put on some worship music or an audio recording of the rosary.

Know that God loves you, is with you, and has a plan for your life! It's hard – very hard – but you have to make your peace with God. And trust that he loves you and knows what he's doing with you.

In all this, my biggest help is my love for the Lord and the continuing experience of his love for me. And so, every day, I want to live out one of his more recent words to me: "Be grateful. And use this to help others. Make love your aim." That's my last piece of advice to you, too.

Family and friends reflect

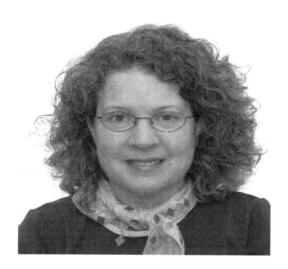

Julie Young recalls her days working for Child and Family Services Adult Day Center which was, for many years, the first and only program of its kind for frail older adults in Washtenaw County, Michigan. She states, "Planning daily activities for participants was constantly challenging, but it was also rich with opportunities for creativity, compassion and humor. I am grateful for them all."

MEMORY OF A POEM

Julie Young

After lunch at the Adult Day Center (ADC), we always planned relaxing activities so the participants could rest or nap for a while. We listened to music, looked at books and magazines, gave manicures and polished fingernails, and played simple word games. I often read aloud – almost everyone seemed to enjoy the jokes in "Laughter is the Best Medicine" from the *Reader's Digest*. For holidays and national days of commemoration I would read speeches, accounts of historic events, and poems to the group. I loved to read aloud and, although it is not a common activity any more, most of the elderly adults at the ADC had read aloud and been read to in school. Quiet attention focused on me while I was reading and, for a short while, I was the "teacher" for this small classroom of special students.

One of those was a petite Hispanic woman diagnosed with early onset Alzheimer's Disease. She was still so young and had beautiful straight dark hair. Her sons had described her as a vibrant, happy person before the onset of the illness – wearing colorful scarves and jewelry, cooking great meals for the family, enjoying music, parties and family gatherings, driving a convertible. One of them said, "She just loved driving that car around…." Now she wore simple clothes – dull t-shirts and slacks. She seemed to be observing everything and all of us but without expression or much recognition. She hardly ever spoke.

On an afternoon near Valentine's Day, I had chosen a few love poems to read to the group. The last one was Elizabeth Barrett Browning's sonnet, *How Do I Love Thee?*. I had to memorize it in high school and still remembered some of the beginning lines and the steady rhythm of iambic pentameter. The meter is simple – one unstressed syllable, followed by one stressed syllable.

I began to read the first line, *How do I love thee?* and just as I was saying the next words, *Let me count the ways.*, I heard another voice in the room begin to recite the poem. As I continued to read this beautiful love poem aloud there was the murmur of each word, repeated by the other speaker, several beats behind the rhythm of the lines I was speaking. It was a soft echo of the poem from a voice I had never heard before. As I read, I glanced up briefly from the book to see who it was, *I love thee to the level of every day's most quiet need*. It was the small dark-haired woman reciting the poem from memory. Her gaze was fixed. She seemed quite unaware of anyone around her. Her words were clear, but spoken only to herself, under her breath. I heard her repeat, *I love thee with a passion put to use/In my old griefs, and with my childhood's faith.* She remembered it all and never wavered or stumbled on line or word. I went on reading the poem to the last line and in the silence when I'd finished, I heard her voice alone, *I shall but love thee better after death.*

She remembered it all and never wavered or stumbled on line or word.

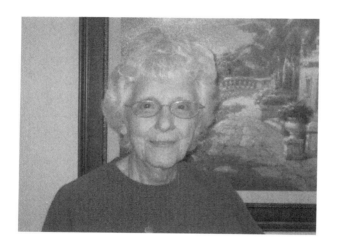

Alberta Sabin writes: "I have lived at the Chelsea Retirement Community (CRC) for nine years. My submission is fiction, but many of the details described in my story are from my experiences with my mother who had severe dementia. Several of my friends at the CRC now live on the campus for residents with Alzheimer's and other dementias. I visit them a couple of times a month and they, too, have influenced my story."

ALZHEIMER'S STOLE MY GRANDMA

Alberta Sabin

I was about 10 years old when Grandma came to live with us. Grandpa had recently died, and we found out from their neighbors that Grandma was leaving the house and getting lost.

Grandma was getting lost? Not my grandma. She was the smartest lady I ever knew. Well, so was Grandpa. He was a smart man. I loved to stay at their house, sometimes for a whole weekend. But that changed when we moved.

We were 200 miles away from them. Because it was so far, we only visited them at Christmas time. But Grandma made up for it. She wrote letters to me. I would write right back and she would too. It was so much fun. I felt like a big girl. I got lots of letters in the mail. None of my friends got as much mail as I did.

And then things changed. She didn't send me any more letters.

Grandma used to be a very good cook. I loved to eat at her house. She cooked so many yummy things. When I visited her, she let me help her. She gave me my very own apron to wear and I got to take it home with me. We would make cookies and cakes, and even bread. That was lots of fun because she let me knead the dough. I got a lot of flour on the table, and on the floor, and on me too. Grandma let me help even when I made a mess but she told me that if you are a good cook, you have to clean up your mess and wash the dishes you used. That was okay with me. I liked putting my hands in the warm soapy water. Grandma would read stories to me and she liked to hear me read to her. Grandpa would tell funny stories. Then we would all laugh. I sure missed him when he died. I cried and cried.

I didn't understand at first why Grandma had to move in with us, but I was very happy she was coming. It wasn't long before I noticed she had changed. She was not the same Grandma I knew.

One night she woke me up and asked me to help her find her bed. She got lost in our house. I couldn't believe it. We didn't have a big house. We didn't have a basement or an upstairs. We had three bedrooms, a bathroom, a living room, a dining room, and a kitchen. Our garage was outside the kitchen door.

When Mom and Grandma and I came home from shopping one day, Mom drove into the garage and we took the groceries into the kitchen. I helped put stuff away. Suddenly Mom looked around and said, "Where's Grandma?"

"I thought she came inside with us," I said.

Mom looked very worried and was looking out the kitchen window. "We have to find her," she said. You look in the garage. I'm going to check the back yard."

I looked all over the garage and she wasn't there. I started to cry and called to Mom, "She's not here!"

Mom was scared. I could tell she wanted to cry too. "Let's go out front. You go this way and I'll go that way. I'm afraid your Grandma is lost. She will be frightened. If you find her, give her a hug and tell her you came to bring her home. Wipe your tears, Honey, and try not to cry."

I walked as fast as I could. I was so afraid we might not find her. All I could think about was that maybe a stranger picked her up in a car and kidnapped her. I saw something like that on TV. I swallowed hard and kept blowing my nose to try to keep from crying.

When I turned at the corner of our block I saw Grandma with a lady I didn't know. I wanted to scream, "You leave my grandma alone." But then I saw that she was holding Grandma's hand and talking to her. I ran up to them and said, "Grandma!"

The lady said to Grandma, "Do you know this girl?"

"I sure do," she said. "This is my granddaughter Bonnie." She put her arm around me and kissed me on the cheek.

"I'm glad to meet you, Bonnie," the lady said as she offered her hand. "My name is Betsy Garth. My daughter Jamie will be so glad to meet you. She hated moving away from all her friends."

That night after supper I heard Mom tell Dad that she talked with Dr. Bromley on the phone. "He thinks Mother should be seen by a neurologist," she said. "He sees signs of dementia. He says we have to be prepared for the time when she will need to be placed in a facility with staff who are trained to work with people who have severe memory loss."

It was all so scary. I ran to my room and buried my head in my pillow. I cried and cried. After a while Mom came into my room. She rubbed my shoulders and hugged me.

"What is going to happen to Grandma?" I asked.

"We are going to take her to a special doctor, called a neurologist, to see how we can help her. You already know that she is not the same person you knew as a little girl. The best thing we can do for her is to love her just the way she is."

The next week Mom took Grandma to see the neurologist. "Your grandma has Alzheimer's disease," Mom told me.

"What's that?" I asked.

"It's a disease of the brain," she told me. "It makes people do things that usually they would never do. Remember how Grandma came to breakfast with her bra on the outside of her sweater? She thought she was getting dressed."

I remembered when she did that. I thought it was funny, then. Now I wished I hadn't laughed. I didn't know that Grandma forgot how to dress herself.

A few weeks later Mom received a phone call. "That was the head nurse at Pleasant View Home. It's a residence for people with Alzheimer's," she said when she hung up. "The director told me they have an opening, and I should bring Grandma to see it and to meet some of the residents."

When Grandma saw it, she thought it was a very nice place, until Mom told her that was where she was going to live. Grandma cried and said Mom was mean and didn't love her anymore. I knew that wasn't true. But I also knew how Grandma felt.

The day Grandma was moved into Pleasant View was a sad day for all of us. Mom said Grandma cried and hung onto her so tight and kept saying she wanted to go home. The nurse told Mom not to worry, that once she got to know some of the residents and got involved in activities, she would be happy and begin to think of it as her home.

Mom visited Grandma every day. Two months went by and I finally got to go for a visit. When I walked into her room, Grandma was all smiles. "Look what I made for you, Bonnie!" She held up a picture of a flower she had pasted on a sheet of paper. On the bottom she wrote, "I Love You."

Alzheimer's stole my grandma from me. She changed. But I know she loves me. And I love her. I always will, even when she doesn't know me anymore. She will always be my Grandma.

The best thing we can do for her is to love her just the way she is.

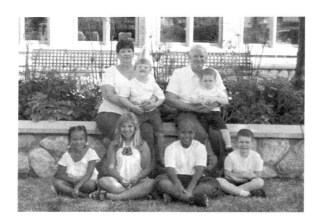

Anita Buckmaster's husband, Rick, was diagnosed in June, 2012 at the age of 61 with younger-onset Alzheimer's. Anita explains, "My mother also suffered from Alzheimer's and passed away almost six years ago. I have written some poetry for family, but never anything to publish. Since Rick's diagnosis, I have had words coming and going in my mind. This felt like the perfect opportunity to put the words into writing and share them with others."

MY HUSBAND IS LEAVING

Anita Buckmaster

My husband is leaving
I don't want him to go
This is so painful
But how can he know?

It began many years ago
On a blind date
It was love at first sight
It had to be fate.

The kids are grown now
It should be our time
This makes no sense
There's no reason, no rhyme

He's been my best friend
Makes me laugh, makes me cry
God must have a reason
I can't help but ask why

My husband is leaving
There won't be another
He's slipping away slowly
As did my mother

Alzheimer's is cruel
The worst of its kind
Who will buy me flowers?
The thought fills my mind

Love each other deeply
Every moment, every day
No looking back, no regrets
Nothing more to say.

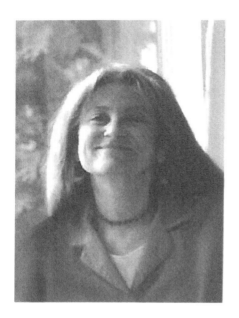

Barbara Tucker is caring for her beloved spouse who has mild cognitive loss following a stroke in 2007. She shares, "We continue to make our way through the uncharted territory of the human mind and the unique opportunities it has brought for enriching our psychological, emotional, and spiritual journey together."

LITTLE BUNCHES OF JOY

Barbara Tucker

"When you scratch my head, I think better all day." It's him, but the words, the voice, are from somewhere else. I have never heard this voice before.

I am astonished. If I'd only known. I well up, regretting all the times I have agreed so begrudgingly, just when I have finally settled into bed, just when there should be no more demands of me that day. And now this tiny glimpse, after five years of peering intently into the opacity of his mind.

This is a different place now — our own private journey. I look back to see we have left our mooring and are floating along in a place where others sometimes venture, but where no one has to stay, except the two of us.

But one where there can be these tiny gifts we give each other — seconds of clarity, born of kindness.

I want it to happen again. My logical mind tries to figure out how. I want another clue. Mine are all exhausted. Well, never mind. No one knows if or when or how, not even me, the expert on my spouse of 27 years.

We have only randomness.

No way to know what completely unpredictable thing will happen next. I am braced for the new trouble it will bring my way.

But I tell myself, "I'm quick, resourceful, up to the challenge."

Nobody is that agile. Or resilient.

What I know now (or is it what I do now?). Control has no value here. Better to let down my guard and experience this life like giving over to a carnival ride. Enjoy the trip through the fun house, where perception may as well be reality.

Not "What the hell next?" but "What precious moments can we find?" Hover above. Watch for them, incubate, foster them.

And pile up little bunches of joyful experiences along the way.

Right after you take very good care to always be watchful to keep in place all the prudent precautions.

"What precious moments can we find?" Hover above. Watch for them, incubate, foster them.

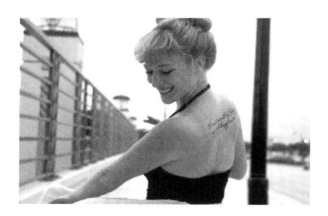

Lauren Scott is a Midwestern whirlwind. She has a BA in writing from Knox College, and is an Interlochen Arts Academy alum. She lives in Chicago where she square dances and has adventures with her boyfriend John. This poem is dedicated to her grandmother, Dorothy Scott.

THE FAWN ENTERS THE WOOD WHERE THINGS HAVE NO NAMES

Lauren Scott

Alice thought, but nothing came of it. 'Please, would you tell me what you call yourself?' she said timidly. 'I think that might help a little.'
'I'll tell you, if you'll move a little further on,' the Fawn said. 'I can't remember here.'

> *(Lewis Carroll, Through The Looking Glass and What Alice Found There)*

Tread carefully. Remember now:
hooves on meadow floors, your mother's tongue;
a fawn's memories must not slip away. How,
at dawn like warm milk, your young bones had sung

of hooves and meadow floors, of someone's tongue
wiping clear the frost settled on leaves. Let this
dawn like warm milk to your young bones, let it be sung
again and again. You must not forget you exist,

your name wiped clear, the frost settled. Let this
image of a fawn persist, snow spots on dark fur.
Again and again, you must not forget to exist
when names fall to earth like rotten berries. Spur

that image you are fond of, persist, dark spots on snowy fur
and—what was it again? Something warm and wet,
its name fallen to earth like a rotten berry. Spur
these memories quickly, run, the wood is dark, forget—

what was that word again?—nothing. Warm and wet
what you can keep within you until dawn.
These memories quickly run. The wood is dark. Forget
your want to know of what you are. Soon, that too will be gone.

Nothing will keep within you until dawn,
no fond memory. It all slips away now.
You know that what you are will soon be gone.
Tread carefully, if you remember how.

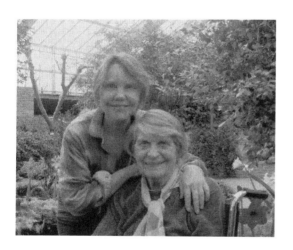

Shari Thompson writes: "Life is full of seasons. Care giving is my season now with my mom living with me. I teach special education in the public schools. My three daughters are young adults creating their own seasons of life. Writing this piece has given me a sense of connection and an opportunity to have conversation with written words. I appreciate the wealth of resources and support our community offers to all of us care givers."

OUR PETOSKY STEPPING STONES

Shari Thompson

Mom held our little girl hands as we walked along the northern shore of Lake Michigan every summer looking for Petoskey stones. Her keen eyes could spot these sparkling pale grey treasures from a distance. We were delightfully excited each and every time we found a stone. When we dipped our fossils in the cool lake water the coral rays glowed like little suns.

Our world was small in those young years of childhood. People knew each other well, there was a sense of connection with family and friends who lived nearby. With time, like most everyone else, we grew up, our worlds expanded; we traveled and started our own families. Mom moved to Florida; Michigan became too cold for her as she got older. On her bedroom dresser she kept a few of our Petoskey stones. Our southern holiday traditions evolved. Spring breaks found us on an early six o'clock flight to Gramma's home in the sunshine and in the pool by noon. Mom's world now had sandy gulf beaches with beautiful shells. She had a good life, working as a nurse, enjoying the pool and her friends.

Five years ago during a visit we noticed some forgetfulness. There was no real concern, her home was full of active grandchildren and there were many distractions. A later phone call from her friend telling us mom brought her toothbrush over and asked for help making a phone call raised serious concern. We got her to make an appointment with the doctor. Watching mom struggle to draw a clock, remember three words, and spell backwards was heartbreak. She was flustered and nervous, she said she had not slept well the night before and that was the reason she did not do well with the questions asked by the nurse. The doctor said she could not drive anymore and would soon be unable to live by herself. Our world changed that day! Mom got angry! The doctor was wrong, she kept saying over and over. She accused us of taking over her life and controlling her. Life became difficult. How do we do this long distance? My sister and I ruminated WHO, WHAT, WHERE, WHEN, WHY? We called these challenges our Petoskey stepping stone decisions. Is there one right decision or several? The world of memory loss was unfamiliar, sad, scary, and emotional.

Our first Petoskey stepping stone decisions involved long distance care. This was short lived – too much worrying, too far away, medications, finances, vulnerability. Our worlds became Venn diagrams, connection evolving to disconnection. Once again we found ourselves on our Petoskey stepping stone, what now? This decision brought Mom to Ann Arbor to live with me. My balance on the stepping stone was becoming more confident. I can say the A word (Alzheimer's) without tears. Another step with Mom led us to the Silver Club, a wonderful place for her to be encouraged and engaged with meaningful activities.

This morning, holding Mom's hand, we walk into the U of M Memory Clinic for our appointment with the neurologist. I watch others coming and going through the clinic doors. Some people push a walker, use a wheel chair, a cane, some smile, others blink, stare, and glance at each other just like me. I wonder how they got here, who are they with, what was their morning like? Did they dress themselves, put socks over their shoes, brush their hair with a toothbrush, put lipstick on their forehead, pour cheerios into their coffee and try to eat them with a fork? Mom did. Our time now to see the doctor. I take Mom's hand and we walk to our room to wait. In comes the doctor, friendly greetings are exchanged. Mom is unable to draw the clock. The questions are asked, Mom smiles, gestures, and says a few unrelated words. When asked to spell world backwards, she laughs as if she is playing a game. I see no anxiety this time. We are told to come back next year. I wonder what life will be at that time.

The steps I take these days are small, redirecting, redoing, and restarting. Mom moves very slowly. At times I enjoy a laugh at Mom's creative sequencing. She is safe and happy. As challenging and consuming as this has been for me, I also am safe and happy. I share my poem with you and a wish for your stepping stone, decision-making journey to be graced with a hand to hold.

Our Stepping Stone World

W   walking when waiting worthwhile wince wholesome winsome warm waterfall wonderful wishful willingness wonder whole why window words weak where wisdom weave welcome weather we windy watching

O   ouch oversee obliging overlap open orbiting outdoors offering observing optimistic obstacle offer old onward oasis oddity odor ocean once overwhelmed

R   raft rambling roundabout respiration relationships rays reasons rearrange radiance rather reflection railway rare receive refresh responsible rhythms roadways recurrent realize ravines resourceful remembering recognizing realm receptive running

L   living losing lost longing lacing leaf listening leisurely lavender laughter light lingering language landscape ladder lasting little local life learning laundry later leading lattice leftovers leaving love

D   daily duty dad display doctor directions dogs diagnosis dessert dancing delicate define daughter decline deciding data dainty drifting diligence detour delicious departure dressing dreamy doze dignity discussion diminish decorate distant distance

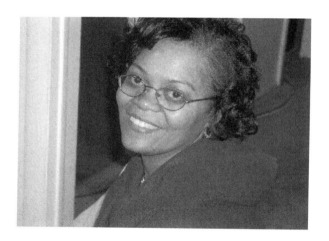

Sharon Greene recently retired from a career of 30 plus years in the Neurology Department at the University of Michigan. Here she writes about her mother.

HERE YESTERDAY, TODAY; NOW GONE AWAY FOREVER

Sharon Greene

My mother was here yesterday, today; now gone away forever

Let me tell you of my mother, Vivadean Alberta Greene. She was the strongest woman you would ever have seen.

She was a lady who used her hands to build anything all over her land.

She was a carpenter you see, and she built houses, speed boats, tables and chairs, wall shelves, wooden docks, and a toy box just for me.

Here yesterday, today; now gone away forever.

She was a hard working mother who had few jobs. First she was a self-taught accountant who maintained the bookwork for my father's first minority-owned business, Greene's Auto Polish and Body Shop in Jackson, Michigan.

Both Mom and Dad were born and raised there yet my mother would be the one to prevail there.

After a long and painful relationship, my dad left us and out went my mother's heart as if it were ripped.

Here yesterday, today; now gone away forever.

She raised three children with my father: one living in New York, Ronald; one in Ann Arbor, Sharon; and one in Jackson, Alvin.

She pulled herself together after many tears that I wiped from her face over the years. She had to make it on her own and maintain her life alone.

She established her own business, Greene's Cleaning Service, and she cleaned doctors and dentists offices all over Jackson for many years. As she dusted, scrubbed, mopped and vacuumed many rooms she began to have pain in her arms, hands, and knees, yet little did I know it was not the pain, but there were white matter changes and atrophy in her brain.

Then little by little small things she could not remember, "Did I take out the trash piled up at the door? Did I set the alarm when I locked the door? Oh my Lord, where are my keys?" These are the words she would say to me. She had such faith in God above and He protected her as His little dove.

Soon she began to get lost while driving and would tell us she was just looking at the trees and shopping for sales at her Goodwill stores. She bought so many things, too many to name, and she would say, "I can't remember why I have this, but it must be for one of my projects."

Here yesterday, today; now gone away forever.

On the weekends I could see the pain was getting worse and this was not a good feeling to me.

I work at the University of Michigan Hospital and fortunately for me it was in Neurology. I took her to the best neurologist there who ordered MRI's on her back that showed severe degenerative bone loss disease. This was in the 1970s. He suggested a small surgery and my mother voiced loudly, "I am not having no surgery; I will just keep taking my SSS tonic."

After many years it was difficult for her to walk and she scooted on the floor to keep from standing on her knees but she kept this from me. One day I came as she crawled to the door, and I said, "Back to Neurology you must go." "What is your doctor in Jackson doing to help you?" I said to her. She replied, "Do I have a doctor here? Oh yeah, I forgot my doctor is giving me pain pills."

She was on high doses of a pain killer, so of course I thought that was why she was so confused; but the pain killer was not the sin, the atrophy in her brain was growing thin.

Here yesterday, today; now gone away forever.

She then saw a doctor and the EMG test was performed. Boy, was my mother mad at me; another painful test you see. The muscles in her arms and legs were wasting away and the bones grew weaker day by day.

Yet another doctor saw her for her memory and he told me things I did not want to hear, but for me it was all too clear. Dementia was taking over her mind, and then things from there were always a decline.

My mother knew from that appointment that she could not hide her problems from me anymore and refused for me to take her so far. "I will get better; you see you don't need to take off work for me. I will take my pills and stay busy with my projects. I think better when I am alone." That was in the 1980s.

Here yesterday, today; now gone away forever.

Her body began to fail and she retired at the young age of 75! She gave her business to her granddaughter Dawn, and the Greene Cleaning Service has another generation of success.

Here yesterday, today; now gone away forever.

My daughter Traci now works for the U of M Hospitals, and we tried again in the 1990s. My mother saw her family doctor, yet to no avail. The story was the same except the dementia now had an awful name; it was the demon disease called Alzheimer's. The stages went oh so fast that it was like a wind storm and only God could calm the sea.

One last attempt was made by my daughter and me to see the best in Neurology. Her local geriatric doctor allowed us to make what we did not know would be Mother's last appointment in 2012 with the neurologist who wanted to try another medicine for Mom, but before I could even get the medicine filled, the demon of Alzheimer's stuck up its ugly head from the bottom of the sea.

She went from hospital to rehab, and finally God said, "Back to the bottom of the sea you dementia/Alzheimer's demon, Vivadean is coming with me." Her great-granddaughter, Taylor, and I put the Christmas tree in her room as her great-grandson, Aaron, rubbed and kissed her head. Taylor asked, "Do you like the tree?" Mother, only able to whisper, said "Pretty."

Mother was placed into hospice. She refused to eat or drink, and was drifting away. Each morning before leaving for work, I crushed her pills and used a syringe filled with Ensure to feed her.

Then finally on that lonely day God gave me hope as she swallowed eight cc's in one, two, and three large swallows without choking or gagging as she had in the previous days. I thought to myself, "Thank you Lord, she is getting better this morning," but the Holy Spirit of reality set in for me as I called the hospice number and asked for a nurse to come that day.

My oldest grandson, Anthony, was with me so I had to fake that I was reporting her vital signs, but I knew God fed her her last intake of nourishment before going on her long trip to heaven into her final resting with the Trinity.

One swallow for the Father, the Son and the Holy Spirit.. Amen. It is well with her soul. Her body was healed as God called her home in the time after I left for work at 7 a.m. and before her caretaker Carmen came at 10 a.m. She passed with only her loving dog Sparkie at her bedside on December 10, 2012 and was placed to rest on December 17, 2012.

As my fiancé, Robert, held my hand while driving from Ann Arbor to Grass Lake, Michigan, he still had hope, but I knew Mother was gone.

Here yesterday, today; now gone away forever.

Her great-grandson, Aaron, rubbed and kissed her head.

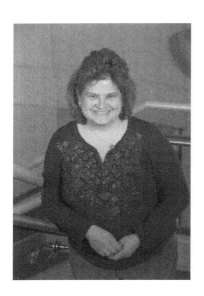

Joanne Lord is a Clinical Research Coordinator, certified by the Association of Clinical Research Professionals since 1999. She is the dementia clinical trial coordinator for the Department of Neurology. Joanne enjoys working with patients as well as their families and plays an active role in all aspects of clinical research. She received her LPN from Marion S. Whelan School of Practical Nursing and her BA from Mount Holyoke College.

THEY DIDN'T TEACH ME THIS IN COLLEGE

Joanne Lord

Some may think goodbye is a simple word, I do not agree. The word goodbye is used millions of times a day. We use it when hanging up the phone, or when someone walks away, a coworker leaves our office, and in hundreds of other situations. I have discovered that the word goodbye is complicated, taking many twists and turns and causing many emotions. They didn't teach me this in college.

The word goodbye has certainly affected me in my career working with patients with dementia, both in Vermont and in Michigan. Some of my most difficult goodbyes involved leaving my job of five years as a study coordinator in order to move to Michigan. I fondly remember one study partner who gave me an angel with purple wings for Alzheimer's Disease to hang in my car. "Why an angel?" I asked. "To keep you safe as you drive from Vermont to Michigan." My angel is still in my car 13 years later!

The goodbyes were difficult because over time I had grown to really care for the well-being of my patients on a personal level, as well as professional. It's hard when they no longer come in, when they pass away, or when a trial is over. And when I knew I was going to be leaving, I wasn't sure what would be the best way to tell my patients goodbye. I knew it was not going to be easy. Would I say the right thing; would I use the right words? Do I tell them goodbye several times on different days and hope they remember, or do I tell them once for the last time and that is the end?

Some may ask why say goodbye to dementia patients when they don't remember? To me, this may be the one time they do remember. And I realized that if they knew I cared about them, that was the most important thing.

After working with patients for so many years, I also got to know their study partners and families. I enjoy talking with families and learning more about them, and getting to know families helps to keep them involved. Some were interested in knowing who I was as a

75

person, just as I liked knowing more about them. I am always happy to share tales of my latest adventures horseback riding, my parents traveling around the country in their RV, or stories about my two nieces.

I became close to two couples over the course of several years. One of the wives, who was a patient, always wanted to know about my riding adventures. She asked the name of my horse. I would always respond, "It's Dusty," and several times during her visit she would ask the same question. I would respond the same way. Never a problem; I would just answer. I put the latest pictures of Dusty and me on my iPod and showed them to her. One day towards the end of the study, she came in all excited and said, "I know his name! It's Dusty." Well, I cried right then and gave her a big hug. She had finally remembered his name.

Another husband and wife in the same study were interested in my latest adventures. Our common interest was skiing. Soon we were comparing Vermont mountains to Michigan mountains, and we decided that Vermont mountains were much better! We always had something to talk about. The patient was losing weight, and I encouraged him to eat more. His wife kidded that she really did feed him.

As the study continued, I realized the patient was going downhill, and it was breaking my heart. I had a hard time seeing a previously vibrant man now unable to speak coherent sentences and unable to recall my name. When the study was over, I was once again saying goodbye and wondering, "How do I do this?" His wife and I both tried not to let the tears fall that day, but it couldn't be helped. They didn't teach me this in college.

I was not sure I would see that couple again. However, this past summer I had the pleasure of visiting them in their home. I was in the area visiting my parents and the couple invited us to their home. It was so wonderful to see them in their own environment. The patient was happy to see me, and once his wife reminded him of my name and where I was from, he did know me. He gave me a big hug as he sat next to me on the couch. He could not converse with words, but his non-verbal skills were sharp and expressed love, gratitude, and knowledge. Once again, tears were in my eyes as I said goodbye.

I look forward to the email messages that occasionally pop up in my inbox when this couple wishes me a Happy Birthday or a Merry Christmas. The last email included a picture of the patient dressed in a Santa suit at the day program he now attends. He had gained a little weight, and his wife was pleased that he actually filled out the suit. I love getting messages from them and keeping tabs on how they are doing. Although it still seems like a goodbye at the end of the email, somehow it brings me closer to them once again, and I wouldn't have it any other way.

I will continue working on dementia trials, building relationships with families, talking about my riding adventures, my parents RV travels, and my nieces. I am also still saying goodbye at the end of trials and at the end of a study visits. I wonder if it will get easier as time passes? As I get older? Wiser? More experienced? I don't know, and only time will tell. Practice can make it easier, but practice cannot make it perfect. Some goodbyes are harder than others. In fact, some are much harder than others. Sometimes the tears are going to come, and I can't stop them. They didn't teach me this in college.

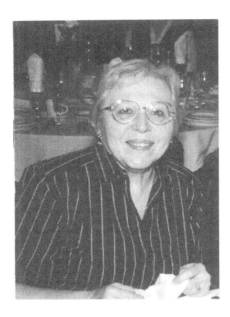

Gail Fromes wrote this remembrance of her mother, pictured above.

MEMORIES OF MY MOTHER

Gail Fromes

My mother developed worsening memory impairments after three strokes over the course of a few years. All of the strokes involved her right brain. This very intelligent woman who once took an adult education course with me in personal accounting and was the first to answer every instructor's question, was now left with cognitive problems that were quite devastating.

When I came to visit her in the evenings at the nursing home, she would ask me what happened at work that day. I would tell her and then 30 minutes later, she would ask "What happened at work today?" Occasionally, she would cock her head to one side, look at me, and then say "Did I already ask that?" I would gently reply that she did, but I would be happy to go over it again and then proceeded to do so. Sometimes, after I started repeating the tale, she would say "Oh, I remember that part."

The hardest experience for both of us would occur when she would ask me to go get my father and bring him into the room. (He had died several years earlier.) I found myself trying to hedge and say he's not around right now, or he had to leave for a few minutes. I then tried to quickly move on to another topic to distract her, but to no avail. Mom would ask again and again until I finally had to tell her that he had passed away. "Oh, that's right," she would say with a look of grief on her face. Because of her memory problems, she had to face the terrible news of her husband's death over and over again.

At other times, her memory was very good, and she remembered the names of people and told stories of the past. She recognized visitors when they came by and often was the only one at her activity sessions who knew the answer to a trivia question. I once told her that a woman stopped me in a store to ask about a good seasoning for roast beef. I had no idea, but when I posed the question to my mother, she replied immediately, "a bay leaf." This was no surprise to me. She was a wonderful chef.

One night, she became very confused and thought I was her sister. She asked me how things were going in New Orleans where her sister lived. I told her who I was quite frequently, devastated that she no longer knew me. Finally, before I left for the night, she recognized me as her daughter and we talked and joked as usual. She died 30 minutes later.

My mother was fully aware of her loss of memory and was very frustrated by it. I was struck many times by the fact that she not only had cognitive problems but had the added hardship of being fully aware that she did. That never stopped her from trying to engage with people and having a positive view of life.

I will always remember her as a woman of great courage who, in spite of three strokes, left-sided weakness, and memory and cognitive problems, always had a smile for everyone she met. She will forever be an inspiration to me.

I was struck many times by the fact that she not only had cognitive problems but had the added hardship of being fully aware that she did.

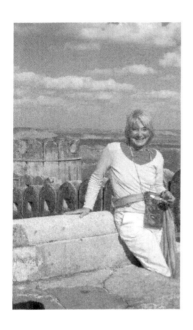

Donna Zajonc writes: "During the winter of 2011, I lived in Tequisquiapan, north of Mexico City. There I renewed my friendship with Hector and met Elizabeth."

HECTOR AND ELIZABETH

Donna Zajonc

From the taxi window, I saw a slightly stooped man walking on the dusty shoulder of the cobblestone road. A straw sombrero on his head bobbed with each step. He was wearing a rough wool vest bordered in black. He was carrying the weight of his world on his rounded shoulders. It was Hector.

Following him was a woman as unsure of her steps as her mind was of its function. The sun bleached the already-faded colors of her blouse and skirt, nearly erasing her from the scene. It was Elizabeth.

I asked the taxi to stop. They were on their way to visit Hector's friend Julio, who lived a few doors from me. They admitted to being tired and eagerly accepted the ride.

Julio had been a friend of Hector's since university days. He became a successful architect while Hector became a professor of literature, a poet, and a dreamer. Julio was one of the reasons Hector relocated from Oaxaca to Tequisquiapan with its quiet, cobble-stoned, bougainvillea-adorned streets.

The other reason was that Hector could no longer live in the house he owned near Oaxaca because his neighbor ran an under-the-counter, over-the-wall auto paint shop spewing toxic fumes which enveloped Hector's patio, seeped through the windows into his house, congested his lungs and reddened his eyes. So he gathered his dogs, Noche and Blanca, one under each arm, and boarded the bus to Tequis where he would benefit from clean air and Julio's warm friendship. In turn, Hector encouraged me to profit from the quiet life and clean air of Tequis. A change sounded exciting. After all, I had been wintering in Oaxaca for 15 years.

It was very shortly after Hector settled into his new surroundings that he received word of Elizabeth's precipitous arrival. Although Hector and Elizabeth's sister had agreed that a visit was a good idea, he belatedly realized that he was speeding headlong into becoming the keeper and caregiver of a needy person for the full month of February having only a small inkling of what she might expect of him.

The friendship between Hector, Elizabeth, and her husband, David, began in Oaxaca, where Hector taught them Spanish. They met with him twice a week, two months a year, for more than ten years. Elizabeth and David had settled into an Oaxaca life of lessons and wintertime friends. To them, Hector was both "maestro" and "amigo."

Now it has been two years since Elizabeth and David enjoyed those days in Oaxaca. David died shortly after their last visit and part of Elizabeth died with him.

A year ago Elizabeth attempted to renew her relationship with Oaxaca where she received the best support Hector could muster. However, she was unable to cope without David and without a good part of her cognitive capacity, and she returned to her California home within three days.

Now, two years later, Elizabeth arrived in Tequis and within days, she and Hector had developed a routine. They would breakfast together and walk to the Vienna Café in the center of the village where they bought cream cakes from a wiry Austrian who made and sold the cakes but never ate them, nor did he lick the frosting from his fingers. When I told Elizabeth the name of the café, she said, "Oh good, I can remember that. I was in Vienna once." At the Vienna Café, Hector would edit his poems while Elizabeth enjoyed the plaza.

Hector kneaded and nudged his poems while Elizabeth circled the square until she remembered Hector. She would hurry to find him and her sense of security. Hector would invite her to have coffee with him. Then they walked around the plaza together, had lunch and later returned to the café where Hector would make further adjustments to his poems while Elizabeth wrestled letters into crossword squares. At some point, she would get edgy and they would walk the plaza one more time, eventually going home for dinner.

Elizabeth's mind accepts new information with great resistance and retrieves old information with even greater resistance. Most often, she can't remember my name or Hector's. That she couldn't remember my name was surprising to me, although it shouldn't have been, as I wasn't a part of her Oaxaca life. For her, I was a new Tequis friend. However, the first time she couldn't remember Hector's name, I was the one confused. She was stumped and frustrated when she tried to remember it. She blurted out, "You know the man I'm staying with. What's his name?" I was shocked. I didn't believe that Hector was the name she couldn't remember.

She was good natured about it and laughingly admitted to forgetting nearly everything. When I told her a friend of mine was coming to visit and that his name was Bob, she said, "Oh good. I can remember that. That's the name of my brother-in-law." She was joyous whenever a name association would help her recall a name or place.

Regularly, Elizabeth and I found things to do together. One day we sorted her money. It seems she and Hector had gone to the bank the previous week and, shortly after, she told Hector that she lost her money. He told her that we have to be more careful, but accidents happen. A few days later, Elizabeth exclaimed, "Oh, look Hector! I found some money I didn't know I had." She agreed that sorting her money was a good plan.

We first sorted the peso notes into denominations of 5s and 10s. Then we stopped to study the picture of Benito Juarez on the 20-peso note. She remembered hearing good things about him. We both were interested in the 100-peso note issued to commemorate the 100th anniversary of the Mexican Revolution. One side featured the railroads (which sadly no longer exist) while the other side featured the valiant Mestizos who brought the revolution to a successful conclusion. We both thought Jose Morales, pictured on the 50-peso note, was very sexy. We found Sor Juana, on the 200-peso note. She was one of the most notable women in Mexican history, ranking in familiarity with La Malinche, the legendary concubine of Hernan Cortes. However, Sor Juana was an ardent nun, a prolific poet and a revered revolutionary.

After sorting, counting and chatting, Elizabeth put her little money, that would be Juarez and Morales as well as the 5- and 10-peso notes, in a little green wallet. She put her big money that would be the Mestizos and Sor Juana, in her big green pouch. Both of which she fit into an even larger green and beige striped carrying bag, which she bought the day she thought she lost her money. Her reasoning was that if she had something big enough to hold all her money, she wouldn't lose it.

On other occasions, Elizabeth and I would take the local bus for trips we jokingly called our trips to nowhere. We took the Number 3 bus, which goes very close to the area where I live. We took the Number 8 bus, which serves the neighboring village of La Tortuga. One day we took the Number 9 bus to the village of San Nicolas. Back in Tequis, we bought a map to see if we could find the villages we had visited and then we'd know we hadn't really been taking a bus to nowhere, but that we had actually gone somewhere!

On days I had Spanish lessons at the Vienna Café with Hector, Elizabeth would go for an amble around the square wearing her sun-faded blouse and skirt. Eventually she would return to confirm Hector's whereabouts.

When my lesson was over, Elizabeth and I would decide on an adventure. One time she bought a small notebook in which she wrote down the places we had visited on our bus trips. She apologized for her handwriting and with a chuckle said, "No one else can read it, but I can."

At other times, we shopped in the local market for food and flowers. When we finished buying everything from calla lilies in honor of Frieda to sweet smelling corn tortillas, we slid the bags and bundles into the back seat of the first suspensionless taxi in the queue and bumped over the cobblestone streets to my house. Once there, Elizabeth washed the strawberries and cilantro and together we'd pick pebbles from the dried beans. We always bought too much of everything, notably cheese. In Mexico, the cheese is good! And Elizabeth had a favorite. She couldn't remember that it was the cheese from Chihuahua that she favored, even when I yapped like a lap dog. She didn't recognize it by sight either, but she did remember the taste. When the lady selling the cheese proffered a bite-sized wedge on a torn piece of banana leaf and Elizabeth tasted it, she smacked her lips. We always bought some, and later we ate it with strawberries while we sat on the shaded patio making words with lettered Bananagram squares. The game, a stepchild of Scrabble, gave us both pleasure and cognitive exercise.

When it was time to draw some letters, I tried to teach Elizabeth to say, "Take five." I'd say, "What do you say?" She would say, "Get some more," with a questioning glance, and I would say, "Take five," and she would smile and repeat, "Take five." When it was the next time to augment her pool of letters, I would ask, "What do you say?" Her face would cloud over a bit and I would say, "Take five." She would smile and say, "Oh yes. I forgot." Even my wiggling five fingers did not help her recall. After one of the failed attempts, she sighed, "Oh, if my students could see me now." Both she and her husband used to be middle-school teachers. A couple more tries and when, once again, I saw her face cloud over, I realized that for her to learn "take five" was not going enhance her enjoyment of the game one iota. I deep-sixed my "take five" initiative.

The days blended together. Elizabeth worked in her young people's crossword puzzle book, while I used the Internet. Then we'd walk to have coffee in the plaza. I brought out the Bananagram squares. We made words. We'd "get some more." She'd smile as she took five. Soon Hector walked by. We'd gossip and joke, share fresh orange juice and listen as the magpies began their late afternoon serenade. Their piercing song was a signal to Elizabeth and Hector that the sun would soon fall behind the surrounding hills. So they hastily left while there was still time for a turn on the plaza before walking home.

For me, Elizabeth was a pleasure, a treat to enjoy at my choosing. For Hector, Elizabeth was a pleasure and a responsibility.

After four weeks, Elizabeth would go home and Hector would be pleased with his effort, exhausted by his experience and apprehensive about what next February might bring.

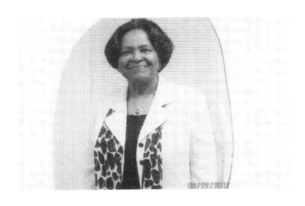

Alvesta Smith wrote in remembrance of her brother, Timothy, who was born on October 7, 1937 and died on October 20, 2008. Alvesta wrote, "Tim's absolute love and joy was his family. He was a loving and devoted husband, father, and grandfather. He lived his life determined and committed to being a good role model and demonstrating exceptional family values. He and his wife, Kathryn, had three children.

MY BROTHER

Alvesta Smith

My oldest brother, Caparton Timothy Evans, lived in Westchester County, New York. Our family who lives in Michigan would visit Timothy and his family from time to time. We would invite Timothy to come over and visit, but he never visited us here in Michigan until he became sick and unable to care for himself. Then we would go over and get him for six to eight weeks during the summer to help care for him. Once when he was around 60 years old, we visited the family in New York during the summer and our brother seemed quite agitated. He had a frown on his face and kept walking around the house. Finally, he went to bed while we were there and that was quite unusual. He would be the one to entertain and take us out to lunch or dinner.

He was a long distance truck driver, driving the truck from Connecticut down into New York City and across the George Washington Bridge into New Jersey. Tim was a dependable and on-time truck driver. The company could depend on him.

When I was a child we lived with our great-grandmother, Ida. She had been a mid-wife for a doctor in Virginia. We lived in the country and some days during the summer my mother would say to me to take Grandma by the hand and walk her almost to the end of the road while talking to her then turn her around and walk her back home. This was for her to get some exercise.

Great grandmother would sit in her rocking chair in her bedroom looking out of the window and see a one-legged man across the forest. I didn't know if he was working, sitting or what he was doing. She never said. But she talked about the one-legged man.

My brother was driving the truck down the New Jersey Turnpike one day and did not remember where he was. A policeman found the truck pulled over to the side of the road, talked with Tim I suppose and called the truck company in Connecticut to dispatch a driver to the New Jersey Turnpike to pick the truck up. Timothy was taken off the truck as a driver but encouraged to help train some of the younger drivers for a while, though he had a number of mini-strokes. Timothy lived for approximately 10 years with dementia.

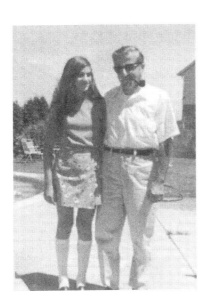

Christine A. Yared is an attorney specializing in employment law, civil rights, and family law, including LGBT law. Her father, Woodrow A. Yared (1916-2004) was an attorney, as well as a district court and circuit court judge. He passed away in 2004, having suffered from dementia during his final years. Christine writes, "I wrote this poem after visiting Dad on August 27, 2004. Dad passed away on November 7, 2004, my mom's 85th birthday."

FATHER

Christine A. Yared

Standing in the final hall
where great minds slip, strong bodies fall.

Black and white photos hung by the doors
illuminate their youth during the Second World War.

In his locked and dreary space,
an empty stare fixed on his face.

As I approached the bed, his eyes lit bright,
I kissed his cheek, then hugged him tight.

I spoke of memories, love and pride,
these feelings and thoughts, to my soul strongly tied.

Tears streaming he cried in his heartfelt way,
"Thank you, thank you," he softly continued to say.

I felt grateful, 'twas not too late,
certain he felt the depth, the weight.

I felt grief, our time was ending,
we both understood, this was my sending.

THE PLAY

Christine A. Yared

(Telephone conversation on a Monday during the fall.)

Daughter: Hello.

Dad: Hi Chrissy.

Daughter: Hi Dad.

Dad: I need your help. Can you help me with a play?

Daughter: A play?

Dad: Yes. I need you to fill a hole.

Daughter: What do you mean?

Dad: I'm working on a play and I need you to fill a hole. Can you help me?

Daughter: Sure.

Dad: Good. You know where we practice, right?

Daughter: I think so, where is it?

Dad: You know, by the park in Cascade. Can you be there tomorrow morning at 9:30?

Daughter: Yeah.

Dad: Good. You should just wear blue jeans, a sweat shirt and tennis shoes because it will be muddy.

Daughter: O.K.

Dad: Thanks, I'll see you tomorrow morning.

Daughter: I'll be there. Bye Dad.

Dad: Bye honey.

At the time of this conversation, my dad was still living at his home with my mom. We knew he was struggling with Alzheimer's or some other type of dementia, but it was all still new to us.

He was still experiencing times when he was living in the present, aware of his surroundings and the events of the day. Of course, with time his condition became worse and it was eventually necessary for him to live in an assisted living home on a locked floor which was for people with similar conditions. At the time of the telephone conversation my dad had started to often talk about the past as if it were the present. When I answered the call and my dad first stated he needed help with a play, I thought he meant a theatrical play since he acted when he attended Ottawa Hills High School in Grand Rapids.

Yet once he added that he needed for me to "fill a hole," I immediately realized he was talking about football. My dad was the quarterback in high school. When I was growing up during the 1960s and 1970s my dad and I would typically watch a couple of professional football games together on Sundays. We would discuss the plays selected and he taught me how to evaluate how they were executed.

When I hung up the telephone, I concluded that he would probably forget about "the play" well before the next morning. Yet I was not certain since I was still learning about the symptoms and patterns of people with Alzheimer's and dementia. Even though it was a work day for me, the next morning I arrived at my parents' house at 9:30, wearing blue jeans, a sweatshirt, and tennis shoes. My dad answered the door surprised and happy to see me stating, "Chrissy, I didn't know you were coming over. Come on in." My mom asked why I wasn't working and I explained that I had some time and stopped by for a visit.

This incident provided a valuable lesson. On one level, his call was emotionally devastating. The call provided evidence that my dad's condition extended beyond forgetfulness or confusion during a conversation. I had to mourn the fact that I would no longer be able to have the type of intellectual discussions that we previously enjoyed. More importantly, this meant that my dad, a retired judge and World War II veteran who was a defense attorney for Japanese soldiers accused of war crimes, was losing his ability to enjoy life by doing what he loved – reading, learning and discussing history, politics, current events, and the events in the lives of those he loved.

Upon further reflection however, the conversation had the proverbial silver lining. My dad was in his element during our telephone conversation. He was working on a productive goal. In his mind he was either a coach or quarterback thinking about the next day's practice, roles that he enjoyed. There was a specific play he wanted to work on and he thought that I would be able to fill a hole which was needed to perfect a play. He thought I could help, located and called my telephone number, explained what he needed and when we ended the call he was pleased that he met his objective.

The telephone call was analogous to a child engaging in make-believe play. For the child, play which is done in a safe, supervised environment is a form of creative engagement which is healthy, enjoyable and educational. As adults we all engage in play in the form of games, hobbies and various social activities. Of course without dementia, we are aware it is play and can move seamlessly between play and the other aspects of our lives.

Yet given my dad's condition at the time, and having witnessed his pain during the times he was acutely aware of his decline, the telephone call and my visit the next day was a brief opportunity for joy. While he was planning the practice, and during our telephone conversation, we were engaging in a form of play that related to an activity we previously enjoyed together. At least during that brief time, he was finding satisfaction and not focused on his disease. Of course, I was also flattered that I was on his team roster.

Another lesson for me was that there is no reason to try to correct a person with dementia who is engaged in a harmless activity or has an incorrect understanding about specific facts. If the activity or words do not create danger or harm anyone, it is valuable to let the person stay in their moment, whether they are coaching a football team or directing a Broadway production of South Pacific.

This experience also allows me to express my wishes should I ever have to live with this disease. If at some time in the distant future, I call you to plan my tennis strategy in my upcoming Wimbledon match against Arthur Ashe, do not tell me that Arthur died in the 1990s or that I have neither the talent nor health to win my assisted-living center's tournament. Instead, encourage me to rush the net and hit to Arthur's weak side.

When you visit me and I think you are President Eleanor Roosevelt seeking my advice about whether we should use a newly developed secret weapon to end the war with Japan, do not waste our precious time trying to convince me that Eleanor was never president. Instead, I will expect you, being the President, to direct your Secret Service contingent to clear my room while we talk.

Finally, be sure to listen carefully and do not presume you already know my advice. My dad was born in 1916 and never wore or cared for denim blue jeans. That telephone call was the first and only time my dad told me that he wanted me to wear jeans.

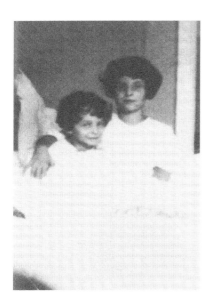

Frieda Morgenstern writes: "As a very private person, nothing short of aiding in an Alzheimer's project would make me want to evoke earlier events in my life. I am a freelance writer, and particularly enjoy doing profiles of people, which I have done for years and continue to do now."

A SISTER'S PERSPECTIVE

Frieda H. Morgenstern

My sister developed Alzheimer's under my unsuspecting eyes. We were always close, through childhood and adulthood, different in our choices of events in our lives, which I attributed to individual preferences. I still miss her very much, or the person I remember so fondly.

My sister and her husband had an extraordinary marriage, so in tune with each other that few friends or outsiders permeated their blissful existence.

After her husband passed away she moved to a retirement community in the Rancho Mirage area of California's desert to be near her son who lived nearby. We kept in touch by emails and phone calls, although her communications were gradually troublesome to me because her son traveled a good deal through his business, leaving her to be dependent on the residents of her facility for companionship. I invited her to visit me in my retirement facility in Ann Arbor – an eye-opening step.

My son, who lives nearby, picked her up at the airport and helped get her settled in my apartment. To show her what my life consists of, we visited such places as shopping areas, the bank, as well as the drug store when she wanted to renew her prescriptions. I introduced her to my pharmacist, whom I have known for many years, so he could give her personal attention. This is when my heart skipped some beats as she drew out of her purse (with great difficulty) a batch of papers that turned out to be copies of her prescriptions. To give her privacy, I shopped elsewhere in the store while she made her purchases. I finally met her in one of the aisles where I found she was doing pirouettes and singing blithely.

Our facility has a community get-together once a week and I introduced my sister to many of our residents. My sister went to the bar, where only wine is served, and there met one of our illustrious Chinese experts to whom my sister attached herself because she evinced an interest in going to China. When this lovely Chinese lady went to her apartment to get some maps and information for my sister, as quickly as possible I came to the rescue, before the fourth glass of wine could be spoken for.

Only a few more instances to make me wonder at the cognitive imbalance my sister was undergoing.

We went to the mall because my sister had always loved shopping. We shopped at different departments, while I asked her to stay at the department where I left her and said that I would pick her up in a short while. When I returned, she was nowhere to be found. I canvassed several aisles, had her name called out on the loudspeaker, finally had the store guard look for her in the store and out into the mall. She showed up, package in hand, cheery and singing in one of the store aisles. My heart was in my mouth.

One day I took her for a ride to show her how lush and green our city is. She looked around, frowned, and finally said, "I don't like this area." Did she miss California sunshine? When we visited my son and daughter-in-law's house she made this tremulous observation "It's too confusing." Were more than two rooms upsetting for her?

When she and I got on the elevator in my building, she delighted in pushing all the buttons, while I cringed. She liked to go down to sit in front of the building so she could greet all who came in or out, though I had told her that no one sits in front of the building except when a car or cab is picking them up.

When she first arrived for her stay, she refused to sleep in the guest room but wanted to join me in the master bedroom where I have an oversized king-size bed. Was she reliving our youth when we had to share a bed? One afternoon as she was napping, I reached over and patted her head, feeling strongly like the big, protective sister that I had always been, but now powerless to know what else to do to help her, beyond submitting to medical know-how.

Sibling affection is noteworthy; when Alzheimer's intrudes it can be devastating.

I will always miss the sister I knew.

My heart was in my mouth.

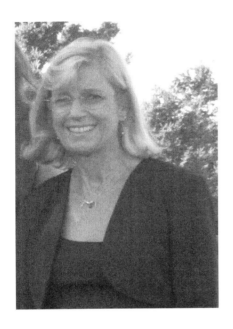

Pam McCombs writes: "My father was diagnosed with Alzheimer's disease in 2004. I have used writing to help me cope. I wrote "Stewart A" originally as an example of a ballad for my first-year writing students. I revised it for the memory loss anthology to help others understand the progression of this disease."

STEWART A

Pam McCombs

Dad/Grandpa/Boppa lives independently
in a facility, with two parakeets.
One yellow, one green that he whistles to
before breakfast, dinner, and supper.

Now, he loves bingo,
eating mixed cheerios
and wearing Hawaiian shirts

Dad/Grandpa/Boppa, born 88 years ago
Stewart A, the twelfth of thirteen,
the youngest son, lived on a farm in rural America.
He grew up watching, catching, and caring for all kinds of birds.

Now, he loves bingo,
eating mixed cheerios,
and wearing Hawaiian shirts

Dad/Grandpa/Boppa joined the Army Air Force in 1941,
was stationed near Chattanooga. He flew many times,
as navigator, across the USA in a B24, but never left the states
because of the Sullivan brothers in WW II.

Now, he loves bingo,
eating mixed cheerios,
and wearing Hawaiian shirts.

Dad/Grandpa/Boppa has Alzheimer's Disease
and doesn't remember what he did two minutes ago.
But, he can play bingo with two cards, goes down to the dining room to eat
and knows his room number 204.

However
Four years have passed and now he is almost 91!
Dad/Grandpa/Boppa only has one bird.
Tammy, the yellow one, he still loves to
whistle to, when we remind him.

He still loves bingo, but has to be reminded.
He still eats cheerios, but doesn't care if they're mixed.
He still wears Hawaiian shirts.

Dad/Grandpa/Boppa has to be escorted to all his meals.
He sits in the lounge watching TV and
sometimes he gets lost going up to room 204.

He still loves bingo, but has to be reminded.
He still eats cheerios, but doesn't care if they're mixed.
He still wears Hawaiian shirts.

Dad/Grandpa/Boppa needs lots of support
to live independently, needs lots of help to remember
when to eat,
when to play bingo,
when to go to bed.
Alzheimer's is slowly eating away Stewart A

He grew up watching, catching, and caring for all kinds of birds.

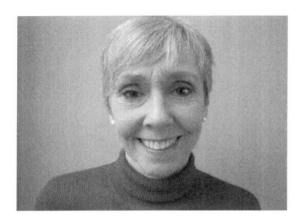

Carol Burton reflects: "As I approach the age of my elder family members and recall earlier years, I often wish I could apologize for the ignorance of my youth and my lack of appreciation for their experience and their fortitude. I am trying to salute them now with occasional memoirs such as this one."

HOMEMADE PHANTOMS

Carol Burton

These days I often ruminate, particularly on the commingling of life and death and memory. In my seventies now, I am experiencing the failures of old age—the losses of body skills and form, interest and desire, the sharpness and detail of memories. No surprise there, beyond the common astonishment that one has actually become an Old Person. How the hell did that happen? Where did that younger self go? What's left?

That's a question of special interest to me because of the dementia-related memory loss in my mother and paternal grandmother, i.e., both sides of my family. I saw the waxing and waning of both these women—what they were in their prime years and at their deaths—and all sorts of existential questions arise. One I'm asking is, what is left of you when you've forgotten everything? What part of one's being is the most immanent, elemental, the last to go?

Grandma was from a German-American community, the first-born in her family. Conjure up a stereotype and there she was—a bossy, large-boned, sturdy woman who worked hard and took her homemaking and her religion seriously. She was masterful in cooking and the textile arts, and her garden was a complex symphony of color and fragrance. Her home was clean, clean, clean and decorated with wallpaper she hung herself, quilts she sewed, and ironed linens with lace edgings she crocheted. She was stout because she also enjoyed the culinary creations that made her "Pa" happy— good farmer food with lots of meat, potatoes and sugar. She was active in her Lutheran church's Ladies Aid Society, went visiting after the services on Sunday, had no use for shyster lawyers, and could tell you what Jesus wanted you to do in all areas of living. I didn't know until I was in my twenties that she was also quite jolly at parties and sometimes downright funny with a woman's grousing kind of humor.

She came to live with my parents after she was widowed, which was a trial for my mother a, shall we say, casual housekeeper, who hadn't been to a church in a long time. Grandma became dangerous in the kitchen, had a child-like fascination with red and hoarded odd red things, took off her clothes in the front yard, and wandered down the country road to "go home." She made little sense in her conversation, which was laced with German and then became nonsense interspersed with stock social phrases like "How's your family?"

So what was left of the woman at the end? I recall a couple things that were perverse expressions of her former self. For one, she cleaned. She tried to wash off a bruise mark on her leg, and she scraped the dark finish off a chair down to the bare white wood with her fingernails. She also liked to socialize. I remember sitting with her in her little room, and she told a good story. It was total gibberish, but her timing and inflection were perfect and her laugh explosive at the punch line. She had me completely engaged, and I laughed heartily and sincerely at the proper time. I never enjoyed her company as much as that afternoon.

My mother lived with my husband and me for several months before she died. It was a trial for us, too. Perhaps the most difficult thing was putting our expectations in reverse. We are both teachers—we work for improvement, and lack of retention is a sign of failure for us. We had to start looking for negative changes in her abilities and not be disappointed when they appeared. Was she just being lazy and avoidant or had she really forgotten how to take pills or flush the toilet? She lost more of her adult self as the months passed, onion-like layers sloughed off, leaving a being who was more childlike, artless.

Some traits persisted as others fell away. I like to think these were the most fundamental and intrinsic parts of these women—the essences that float about in our recollections and analyses of them. For my grandma it was nourishment, work and social interaction. Her appetite finally yielded to her illness, but otherwise she enjoyed all things with food—preparing, offering, and eating. She had a strong sense of rightness about how a house should be run, how people should behave, and how hard work was necessary to that rightness. She kept her hands busy and talked, talked, talked. That was what she was to the end—busy hands and something to say.

For my mom it was laughter, personal beauty, nurturing, and naughtiness. Her naughty streak was there from childhood on, according to the family legends. Not meanness or criminality—mainly bedwetting, lots of beer, and dirty jokes. She lived thirty years as a widow in the country and always had a huge variety of company of all ages. She was an easy touch and people took advantage of her hospitality and good nature, but they also checked up on her and just adored her.

Things she loved until the end—colors, windows with scenery, nature shows on a non-stop television, looking pretty, jokes, and me. Although she couldn't remember my name, she did know that I was her Baby. In her last hours she smiled vaguely when I told her I was going to curl her hair and when my husband asked his daily silly question, "Would you like a kiss, Madam?" And when I told her she could let go, within two minutes she died. Here was this shell of my mother, unable to call up anything from her body or mind, and yet she was still there and is still here with me now. I don't know how else to say it. Not breath or heartbeat, but something of her nature persists playfully beside me. Hi, Mom.

I look at scraps of paper they wrote on—lists, recipes—and handwork they did and I am just so regretful that I was too busy to siphon off their thoughts and memories while they were still accessible, too callow to appreciate how many thousands of stitches and meals and gifts and love notes made up these women. I'm left to distill them into phantoms that I carry in my head, that I talk to as I drive, that I embellish as I approach their final ages and understand them so much more.

And I wonder how I will be remembered, how I want to be remembered, how to create my own ghost.

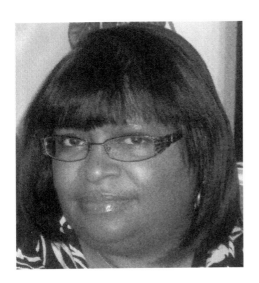

Deb Mecks is a married first-time grandmother with two grown sons. She is a temporary administrative assistant for the University of Michigan Health System. Deb received her BA in Journalism from Wayne State University ('87) and is applying to the U-M master's degree program for the study of Creative Writing.

WHERE HAS MY LOVE GONE

Deborah Mecks

My husband was driving as we glided down the I-75 freeway headed to a branch of my mother's credit union in Lincoln Park, Michigan. My mom was in the back seat. "Where are we going?" she asked again for the fifth time.

Patiently and respectfully I answered her for the fifth time, "To the bank, Mom, to get the power of attorney papers notarized."

"Oh," she responded.

I knew she didn't remember why we were going to get power of attorney papers notarized, which is precisely the reason why we needed to get the papers notarized. Mom had been diagnosed with dementia one year prior. She kept the diagnosis to herself until she could no longer handle her day-to-day business without my help. I had been joint on her bank account for years. Now I had taken over paying her bills, but I needed to legally have her power of attorney so her creditors would give me confidential information about her accounts.

The inertia force from the car climbing up the Rouge River bridge forced me to sit back in my seat. I bobbed my head to the music coming from the radio. I wanted to sing but couldn't because I was trying to hold my breath so I wouldn't inhale Southwest Detroit's distinct smell — a mixture of gasoline and burnt rubber. "Where are we going?" Mom asked again, this time with more curiosity. She must have smelled it too because when I turned around and looked at her I laughed because she had her nose scrunched up. I answered her yet again, "To the bank to get the power of attorney papers notarized." I had to talk loud because her hearing was failing also and she refused to wear her hearing aids. "This don't look like the right way," she said as she looked out the window at the skyline filled with factory chimneys blowing out stinky factory smoke.

I continued to study her wondering, how could this frail little lady sitting in the back seat of the car dressed in a frumpy pink jogging suit and dirty sneakers be my mom? Just two short years ago she was a maverick. A fashionable maverick who would have never been seen outside in a frumpy pink jogging suit or dirty sneakers. As a matter of fact, after we handled our business at the bank we had to stop by Dietrich Furs, in Detroit's New Center area, to get her mink coats out of storage.

I was getting a crook in my back as I studied her from the front seat. We were going down the bridge now so I straightened up in my seat and looked out my window while humming to a song on the radio still pondering to myself, how could this be the same woman who was a much respected church musician whose choir members called her The General behind her back because she was such a perfectionist. Now here she was questioning me about where we were going and why, like my sons used to do when they were children.

In 1963, my mom divorced my father because of his unforgivable behavior. Well, she could have forgiven him, but she felt life is too short to be dealing with his mess, and she sent him packing back to his mother's house. Three years later she bought a nice two-bedroom house with a remodeled attic on Detroit's northwest side. This was unusual behavior for a woman back in the 60s, especially a Negro woman. Most women of the day, especially minorities, got married and became housewives. They didn't have their own money, they were not extended credit or financing, and they dealt with the drama that their husbands threw their way. But my mother had a good job teaching music in the Detroit public school system. She was a role model in a time when the second wave of the women's movement was just beginning to swell.

Mom commenced to raise my sister and me as a single mother. She provided us a middle-class lifestyle without the help of social services. I never missed a meal and our school clothes came from Hudson's (now Macy's) and Saks Fifth Avenue. She was the perfect role model for me as I found later in my life I would need to make my own way as a divorced single mom. I am not boasting. I want you to understand that the woman who raised me and my sister, and the woman who I am now giving care to, are two different people.

The initial reaction of my family to my mother's dementia diagnosis was panic. She is the eldest of five siblings, and they were not used to her not being on top of her game. It also became evident that Alzheimer's/dementia was a family illness that we all would be dealing with in our senior years. My great aunt and one of my mother's brothers suffered from dementia before they made their transition. In an attempt to try and find answers on how to deal with her illness I signed up to do the Alzheimer's Walk at the Detroit Zoo in the summer of 2012. I had fun at the event but trying to rally people was not a rewarding experience. The family I expected to be all in with me, wasn't. Oh well, live and learn. I still get the Alzheimer's email newsletter to keep up with medical information.

After Mom was diagnosed she immediately became my responsibility. She has one brother that lives in Detroit and the rest of our family members live in New Jersey or California. I love my mother and I would not trust anyone else to take care of her. I squeeze in checking up on her between being a wife and an employee. My sister, who lives in New Jersey, is concerned but can't help me, so my husband is my tag team partner.

In the beginning, my non-Michigan family members would call me in a panic when they would call Mom and she didn't answer the phone. They immediately thought something was wrong and would beg me to drive from Westland to Detroit to make sure she was not sick, hurt, or dead. With gas prices being high, me making that fifty-mile round trip every time they got nervous soon became unfeasible, especially since they were not sending me any gas money. So, I immediately had to let them know I would not be speeding down to Detroit on a whim anymore. My husband and I visit her twice weekly and call her in between visits. Once I explained to them that Mom didn't answer the phone because she simply didn't want to talk, they calmed down. They didn't like it, but they calmed down.

With that under control, now we worry about her driving. In the beginning of her diagnosis she drove everywhere even though she has bad hearing and cataracts in one of her eyes. I took her to the doctor and he said the cataracts were not ripe enough to remove, and if she felt comfortable driving then she should drive. I don't agree with him, and my family wants me to take her keys. I, on the other hand, think the Secretary of State should do its job and deny her license renewal this year. I emailed SOS and asked what test they have in place to make sure seniors are still healthy enough to drive. In short, they explained that if she doesn't pass the eye test then she won't be getting her license.

To make my life easier, I am now about to move my mother into a unit in my condo subdivision. She doesn't have enough money to go into senior housing. When we first mentioned moving her a year ago she refused. Now as the dementia takes over I think she is welcoming the idea. My husband and I were thinking of moving to a bigger condo or renting a house, but the thought of packing up two houses and then loading it all on a truck left a nasty taste in our mouths. Besides, I think it will work out better having her own place. That way when family comes to Michigan to visit her they can stay at her place and visit for as long as they want.

So, as the three of us glide through life together I don't know if I'm doing everything right, but I am doing the best I can to keep Mom happy. I've made it a point to tell my sons to get them prepared for the day when they will have to care for me and their stepfather. My boys taking care of me? Oh geez! I better start getting myself prepared mentally.

I want you to understand that the woman who raised me and my sister, and the woman who I am now giving care to, are two different people.

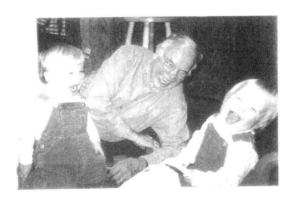

Katherine Stribe shares: "Since the time that my husband Ralph and I heard he had Alzheimer's, we decided we would talk about his condition openly with people. Thus, here is the Christmas letter I wrote in 2010 to family and friends."

GOOD NEWS/BAD NEWS

Katherine Stribe

The bad news is Ralph is declining in his Alzheimer's.
    The good news is he has kept his pleasing personality.

The bad news is Ralph can't understand the commentators on TV.
    The good news is we enjoy watching Bill Cosby and other comics.

The bad news is Ralph can't put words together to join in conversation.
    The good news is he loves having people around.

The bad news is Ralph doesn't do woodwork anymore.
    The good news is he goes to Silver Club where he paints, sings, and
    has lots of fun.

The bad news is Ralph's knees and shoulders give him pain.
    The good news is he doesn't mind doing the exercises to
    strengthen them.

The bad news is our traveling days are over.
    The good news is we can go to plays, concerts, and grandkids' flag
    football, softball, and basketball games.

The bad news is Ralph has to put up with me doing all the driving.
    The good news is he tells me I'm a good driver!

The bad news is Ralph can do little for himself.
    The good news is he tells me he loves me and he appreciates all
    that I do for him!

The bad news is we don't do a lot of talking.
    The good news is we do find a lot to laugh about.

The bad news is Callie's family and many of you live far from us.
    The good news is we have Andy's family, neighbors and friends
    around here who give us lots of support.

Medical students creatively interpret

Reprinted with permission from Club Member, Silver Club Programs, U-M Geriatrics Center

Now a third-year medical student at the University of Michigan, Shilpa Gulati recounted her experience after meeting with a member of a memory loss program.

TALKING TO JUNE

Shilpa Gulati

When I first meet June, she is glowing. Unadulterated excitement dances across her face as we exchange the most routine pleasantries and begin to scout out a room for our interview. The Center reminds me of my kindergarten with wooden tables and chairs, colorful walls, and sing-song voices echoing down the halls. As she tells me about her favorite group activities, her lips stretch out into an indiscriminate smile, her default expression, her child's pose.

A distraction hurries past us and June pauses with the hint of a lost thought. We share a moment of confusion before she turns to me, eyes searching for a reminder of our previous direction.

I take her hand and we move down the hallway again slowly, because June takes small, steady steps. A strip of tape is lobbed over the door jamb into the game room so we don't have to turn the handle; these senior-friendly measures are embedded throughout the center, unannounced but conspicuous.

We take seats around a wooden card table. I ask her about her daily medications and the routines that help her maintain the remnants of her independence. I learn about how irritated she feels when she has to rely on others. She shows me her Alzheimer's bracelet; if she is lost and then found, this has instructions to return her home.

As we skip between subjects, June's attention undulates. I can't detect any discernible change in her expression; her pupils might dilate, or maybe her wrinkles relieve by a millimeter or two. She's there and she's not, in an instant, with no warning.

June has a husband, a retired construction foreman who takes good care of her. When she met Karl, he was a customer at the diner she worked at, and while she didn't know about her Alzheimer's yet, she could sense something was wrong. I cringe reflexively at this, the beginning of a devastating disease overlapped with getting to know the love of her life. I feel even guiltier when I notice that June is still smiling.

"I'm happy though, you know?"

The program coordinator knocks and drops her head between the door and the jamb, slowly drawing it back to reveal a stocky gray-blonde man, the prototype of a lumberjack. "June? Karl is here to pick you up."

June's taut lips collapse into dry folds as she draws them into a frown. "That's not Karl."

There is a silence, broken moments later by her innocent giggle. "I'm kidding! Hon, we're having so much fun, can we have a couple minutes more?"

June turns back to me to confide: "He's an angel."

"I'm happy though, you know?"

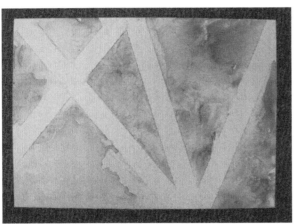

Reprinted with permission from Club Member, Silver Club Programs, U-M Geriatrics Center

Jonathan Awori is an Assistant Professor of Theatre and second-year medical student who composed this poem after completing a class assignment to interview a member of a memory loss program.

PIECES

Jonathan Awori

Hippie. Aneurysm. Collage. New Haven. Santa Fe. San Francisco. Ann Arbor.

I can't remember really anything to tell you.

Communist. Webster's Dictionary. Latin. French. Aneurysm enlarges.

What do you get out of your art?

No one has ever asked me that before. It satisfies a deep need…. I'll write that for you; here, let's use this bright paper…. I saw her words in her handwriting and caught a glimpse of that need.

My father never left the communist party. They made him leave his job as a professor and then he went to work for Webster's dictionary defining words.

The irony. That a man sidelined by a label, a single word "communist," should move on to defining words. His daughter, Mary, inherited his penchant for language, studying Latin and French. Aneurysm grows even bigger.

I wish you were here every day; I'd remember more stuff.

Had she really forgotten?

Do we really have memory loss or is our memory only misplaced, waiting for the most unlikely of triggers, a medical student on a fall afternoon asking a few questions?

Mother. Died. High school education. Father professor. High school diploma versus PhD. You know how that is. When Mom died, that's when I started making art. She always used to make art. She made art all the time, but Dad was a reader and a thinker. So you know….

Did you start studying art to connect to your mom?

That's a nice thought, but really, I think it was about trying to figure out who I was.

Bachelors. Masters. Doctorate. I never did anything with them . . . .

Why San Francisco? I was a hippie . . . followed some man probably . . . aneurysm about to explode . . . .

Look at my cards . . . I like to use different textures.

What do you want people to get out of your art?

I hope they like it.

Aneurysm explodes . . . life in fragments . . . thoughts in pieces . . . exploditus . . . mahemium . . . reperio . . . detoner . . . grabuge . . . decouverte!

Who am I?

Starting again . . . l, l, l, lear-nn, --ing e-e-e verything.

Aneurysm rupture, the stats: 1/3 dead; 1/3 vegetables; 1/3 make it. I'm one.

What is your favorite kind of art?

Collage.

And that made perfect sense. Mary's life, a scattered, scintillating journey before the aneurysm rupture was even more diffused after the event. Now she puts the art pieces together, facing different directions on the cards she creates, each piece an incomplete part of something else, making no sense on its own.

But when she lifts up the completed card to show me, there is a precarious coherence, a fragmented beauty, a life still being lived . . . and forgotten . . . and remembered.

I wish you were here every day; I'd remember more stuff.

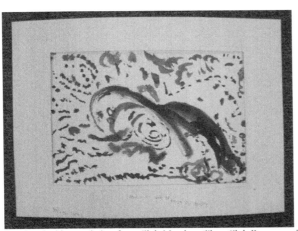

Amanda Wong is a second-year MD/PhD student at the University of Michigan Medical School. This piece was written based on an interview generously granted by a member of a memory loss program. Amanda imagines herself as the son, a physician.

UNCONVENTIONAL ART

Amanda Wong

"What are you listening to there, Dad?" My dad was sitting at the kitchen table, with ear buds in his ears, fidgeting with some black, pocket-sized device that looked like an audio cassette player. I figured maybe he had dug up his Walkman, out of nostalgia, to listen to old tapes of his. He often used music to get him in the mood to do what he did these days to pass the time, which is what he had done, and made a career out of, his whole adult life – that is, making "unpopular art." Those were his words. "I am a creator and purveyor of unpopular art," he would declare.

With all of my dad's talk about unconventional art, and his recurrent monologues on the importance of producing art that provides commentary on the social and political issues of the day, one could mistake him for being part of the generation that came of age during Woodstock and the Civil Rights movement. But the 60s and 70s were actually a time when he was working for a commercial art company, while I was growing up. These days, when reminiscing on my teenage years, I often feel, with a twinge of regret, that my dad was born a generation too soon, and that it should have been he rather than I to have been young during those times.

Still, Dad has no dearth of stories to tell from his own childhood. He was born in the year 1930, the year after the Great Depression had started. To this day he can relate with great clarity stories from his past – of the effect the death of his older brother had on him in his childhood; of his chance to visit the North Pole while he was stationed in Alaska during his service in the Korean war; and with the most vivid detail, of the day he met his wife, my mother, and the days they passed together until 18 months ago when she passed away. It's just the more recent stuff, like what he had for breakfast this morning, or where he misplaced the iPod I got him for his last birthday, the short-term, trivial stuff, that recently has had a hard time sticking.

"I'm not listening to anything," my dad answered grumpily, still playing with the device. "I haven't been able to hear anything since my hearing aid got stolen."

Oh no, I thought, he had lost something again. Next it was going to be his bifocals, and he'd be at his art deaf and blind. Truly unconventional. The contraption he was holding, then, must be some sort of replacement hearing aid. "Is that what you got to replace it then?" I asked, ignoring the fact for now that the hearing aid he lost was a $900 premium hearing aid that my wife, Barb, and I bought him after he had come back from the doctor six months ago saying that his doctor recommended that he get one. "Yeah. My hearing aid was stolen," my dad repeated. "Hearing aids are too damn expensive, so I went down to the Radio Shack and bought myself this piece of crap. It's a Stereo Amplifier Listener. Got it for $26.99," he said, with a mixture of pride and disgust.

Who would want to steal your hearing aid, was what I wanted to say. But not wanting to sound like I was accusing him of lying, I asked instead, "Are you sure you didn't just misplace it somewhere? Have you looked around for it?"

"No, because it was stolen. It was Hilda." Hilda was my dad's home nurse aide.

"That doesn't sound like something Hilda would do," I responded. "Have you checked your bedroom?"

"Hilda's a great gal and all, but hearing aids are expensive. Her parents are hard of hearing too."

This took me a second to process. "So you're saying Hilda stole your hearing aid so she could give it to her parents?"

"That's right. Hilda stole my hearing aid, 'cause her parents needed one. So now I'm stuck with this piece of crap."

Which parent would Hilda end up giving it to, I thought to myself. She'd have to choose favorites between her mom and her dad. Maybe they'd share the stolen, prized hearing aid. But because he seemed content playing with his new Stereo Amplifier Listener, I left my dad alone.

Usually I tried to take Dad's memory loss lightly, to view these incidents with bemusement, rather than concern, which was the approach my wife took. It was only after her urging, in fact, that I had asked my dad to move in with us last year. Barb and Dad had always gotten along, which was a good thing. I was grateful to never have had to negotiate the nasty politics that normally plague the relationships between spouses and in-laws. But sometimes I felt guilty that maybe Barb cared about my dad more than I did. Or at least that she had the appropriate emotional response to his symptoms of memory loss, instead of the colder, more objective one inspired in me. As a doctor who took care of patients with much later stages of dementia, I knew that the memory loss my dad was experiencing put him at most in a mild stage of Alzheimer's disease. Sometimes it is difficult to determine whether patients who display mild symptoms – having trouble recalling recent events or conversations, for example, or demonstrating forgetfulness about where one has placed objects – actually have Alzheimer's disease.

I knew that Dad wasn't just "getting older," which is the diagnosis patients often prefer to hear. But a part of me couldn't help rooting for him, for his mental prowess, to hold on for longer. As with most things in life, perhaps part of this was out of self-interest. There is some component of genetics that comes into play in acquiring neurodegenerative diseases, and so rooting for him in part meant rooting for myself.

My dad, who had stepped out of the kitchen a few minutes before, came walking back holding a different object in his hands. "Hey son, take a look at what I found," he called.

"Your hearing aid?" I supposed hopefully, though I knew in all likelihood it was not. My dad was a stubborn man, not one to openly admit to mistakes. Had he actually found his hearing aid, he probably would have simply continued using it without ever mentioning that he had found it. Such an utterance would implicate him in an act of forgetfulness that he, like I, preferred to overlook for the time being.

Ignoring my comment, or perhaps not hearing it – it was always hard to tell which was the case – my dad handed me a picture frame. Inside was a photo taken from when I was a little boy. It was of me, my dad, and my mom standing next to a sculpture my dad had created for a public library in Louisiana, where we had lived during my childhood years. The structure featured a couple of children admiring a spiral of books. For a man who boasted about specializing in unconventional art, my dad had made a lot of conventional pieces.

But maybe that was the point. That one must understand what makes art conventional before reimagining it into something unconventional. In fact, as his son, perhaps I was guilty of committing the opposite crime. In spending my days in an academic medical center taking care of patients with the most complicated, unusual, and unconventional of conditions, I seem to have missed, or chosen to miss, a strikingly conventional case, in one of the most important people of my life, standing right in front of me.

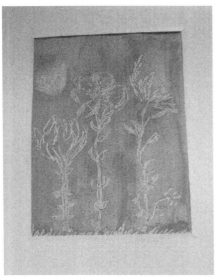

Greg Jaffe, a second-year medical student, stepped in to the first person role in his fictionalized remembrance based on an interview conducted with a female member of a memory loss program.

EVERGREEN

Gregory Jaffe

I used to make 'em carry me. Faked 'em out all the time. This was back when I was a child in a place called Evergreen, Alabama. I grew up on a farm where we grew stuff, mostly corn. I was the youngest, you see, the baby of the family, and my siblings wouldn't let me work; they were afraid I'd mess something up. But at the end of the day I'd pretend I was tired, and I'd go to cryin' too, and make 'em carry me. I'd ride home on their backs.

I used to work over at the museum, I was a supervisor. Kids would always be reachin' out and getting fingerprints on the glass on the paintings, things not to be touched. My job was to keep 'em clean. Worked there for six years. People used to ask me, "Why a museum?" I just liked the pictures, I guess, thought they were really nice.

The things that are important I put on a "don't forget" list. Taking pills, going to doctor's appointments, paying bills. And if I forget things, it doesn't bother me much cuz if it's not on the list, it must not have been important!

My friend Thelma introduced us, my husband and me. He liked to dance, and I liked to dance too. He always had this look on his face like he was up to no good, causin' some kind of trouble. My how we used to dance, practically 'til the sun came up.

I live with my daughter and her husband out here now. I'll tell my daughter I can move out soon, go to live in a retirement community. She says to me softly "Oh Mom, don't do that." What a nice girl she is.

I've got what they call a delayed memory—I'll remember something just a few days later. I've got a trick, though. The things that are important, I put on a "don't forget" list. And it don't bother me much if I forget something, cuz it must not have been important!

Obituaries? I don't keep 'em around. Want 'em out of my mind. If they lying around, they bring back too many memories. I don't really know dates either; I can just say it was a long time ago.

I'm headed out to Pensacola in a week to visit my sister Clemmy. I've got lots of nieces and nephews out there, but they all grown now. I used to live out there when I was a teacher; I like living up here more though, like the quietness of the place.

I'm what you call a "retired person" now; used to work in the big museum. Six years I worked there, made sure the glass covering the paintings was clean. Kids always be touchin' the glass, getting fingerprints on 'em. I was a supervisor, you know.

I remember the call, came 'round midnight: "Ma'am you got to come down to the emergency room, your son has been in an accident." He was out with his friends, hit by a man who was drunk. I don't like talkin' 'bout that much though.

I'm the baby of the family. Had five brothers and sisters: Clemmy; Edna; Erma; James; and Harry. I'm headed down to Pensacola soon, haven't really been down there since Clemmy passed. The weather down there is real nice this time of year.

The things that are important, I put on a "don't forget list".

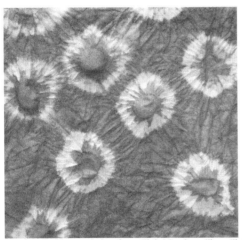

Thomas Filardo, a second-year medical student, wrote this reflection based on a class-assigned interview.

KAREN

Thomas Filardo

In his essay, *The Lost Mariner*, Oliver Sacks writes about a patient of his who was, for all intents and purposes, stuck in 1942. This man is incapable of forming new memories and begins each day anew without any memory of the events of the preceding decades. And even within each given day, he cannot hold a conversation or task for very long. Sacks is dismayed to realize that in this man, he sees a lost soul, a person completely without an identity in the present. Through his story, Sacks makes us look into ourselves and ask: without memory, what am I?

It is in this context that I think about Karen.

Karen is a delightful woman in her 60s. I sat down and talked with Karen and her husband, Mark, a long-haired man with a more reserved, if not unfriendly, air. We were meeting at the Center where Karen was a member of a group for those struggling with memory loss. Karen's hair framed her face and she smiled at me with a familiar kindness through her reading glasses.

With her easy air and exuberant personality, Karen is perhaps not the first person who would come to mind when you think about memory loss. But in the first moments of our discussion, it was clear to me that something was going on. For Karen, the details just won't seem to crystallize. When she tried to answer a question like "How long have you and Mark been married?" or "How long have you lived in the area?" the glow of the memory – the person, the place – could be called to mind; that diffuse, pillowy cloud of emotions is untouched. But what Karen could not seem to do was drill down and gather the details without help.

Karen therefore described most everything from the recent past in the vaguest terms. When asked about a certain person in her life, they were invariably "wonderful." Without prompting, Karen couldn't remember the couple's recent trip to Montana to the part of the state dotted with lakes made by glacial movement. It is an annual trip they have made for more than a decade, after a cross-country drive once happened to take them through the region. And while she remembered that the recent trip was very relaxing and that the scenery was beautiful, she couldn't tell me about anything the couple did in particular without her husband's help. Except for how delicious the ice cream was. Apparently the couple ate a lot of ice cream on their vacation.

Karen worked for many years as a nurse. When I asked what kind of work that entailed, she answered simply, "I helped people." I asked her if she could be more specific, maybe give me an example of a specific patient she helped or a memorable day on the job, but she passed by the question. She insisted, "It has always been my job to just help people who were in need."

I guessed that it had come time to ask the difficult question I had been preparing, and Karen's work gave me a clear avenue in which to ask.

"So I would imagine you have worked with a lot with people who have suffered from memory loss. Can you tell me what it's like to have difficulties with your memory?"

Karen didn't react differently to this question than the others. And while her smile didn't falter, it did sadden. "I don't." She started again, "No. I don't think I have any memory problems." Mark pointedly looked away.

I was surprised, and quickly changed the subject. I noted that every time Karen would hit a block in her memory and struggle during our conversation, Mark would help her by providing the "jog" for her memory. And in each of those moments, Karen was not thinking, "Why can't I remember these things?" but instead treated each omission as something that was on the tip of her tongue, a natural little blip of forgetfulness isolated from the others.

The lost mariner is admittedly an individual in a much different scenario than someone like Karen. However, what she seems to have lost is the ability to integrate the details of her daily life. The details of her present, things we take for granted as guiding forces, the things that imbue our daily activities with direction, are inaccessible. But it was clear that I had not gotten the whole story, for Karen exuded the confidence of someone for whom their purpose in life is still firmly cemented in place.

I dug further. "Karen, what do you like about coming to the community center?" She said, simply, "I'm here to help." To Karen, her role in the group is the one she has always taken on; she is a helper. She volunteers her time to do what she knows best – what she has done tirelessly for her adult life – which is to work with older folks who could use some support. And perhaps this is the best explanation for why Karen denied that anything is wrong – at the core, with the aid of a solid support system, her purpose in life – to help – remains untouched by illness.

In all of this, it was easy to focus on the limitations in Karen's memory. But to the contrary, in the short period we spent together she revealed to me a lifetime worth of memories, the kinds of things that shape a life in a way nothing else can. She remembers her marriage to Mark, 10 years after they met. A wedding which for he, a professional chef, busily organized the food preparation during their wedding reception. They still joke that she was alone in far too many of the pictures, including the one of her tasting the first bite of wedding cake. She remembers taking the train from Detroit to Chicago with her mother as a child, and how the sound of the train rattling through her neighborhood at night filled her dreams with a sense of adventure.

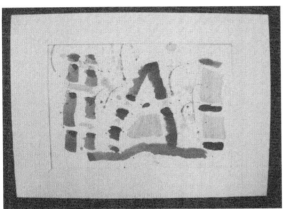

This poem was conceived of after Brittani Jackson, a second-year medical student, interviewed a memory loss group member.

THE ONES LEFT

Brittani Jackson

We are the waking men.
We gaze through one-way glass with wide eyes.
We watch you stir on the other side of us
With dried up words.
The timer runs but do not be roused from your good sleep
It is our alarm. Not yours.

We are the waking men.
Shaking men.
Prodding, pulling, pleading men.
We rise through sundown.
To rock you, hold you to our heart and
sing haunting lullabies into the caverns of your ears.

We are the sleeping men.
Frantically searching for cover
from the daylight streaming in through dirty windows.
Wrapped up in cozy dreams
that no longer seem familiar.

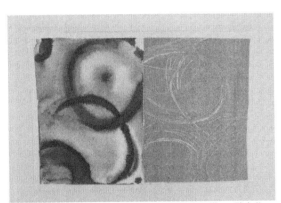

Emily Smergel, a third-year medical student, wrote this piece after interviewing an individual living with memory loss. Reflecting on the interview, and then thinking about the writing process with one particular person in mind, brought forth the idea of how disorienting it might feel to not remember. She wrote the piece with that in mind.

THIS IS YOU

Emily Smergel

You were nervous. Almost shaking. Were you anxious about revealing your story? Worried that you would forget key events in your history? Tense because we were strangers with you in an unfamiliar place?

When you spoke it was faint, but you were solid. "I was diagnosed with dementia. I have dementia. One of the questions I wanted to ask was how you get it...and then I found out that it can run in families. And now I'm here."

You worked for years organizing, keeping track of things, and being responsible for remembering. Your intonation and pauses hinted that you must have known something was changing. You said that you had to write things down (you still do). Dementia skipped a generation; your grandmother had dementia. Does that connect you to her? You remember spending time with her when you were 10. And you remember not understanding why she would repeat herself. A diagnosis did not exist until later.

"My father raised us girls to work hard. Get a job. Take care of yourself. Be independent, because he might not do it for you." You had a good childhood – playing on the beach, picnics, strength, morals, determination. You are number two of five girls and one boy. When you spoke of your father's death you had that sense of sadness that occurs right before tears. You miss him. Details of that day must still be clear for you; you remember being in the hospital. You were a little girl when it happened, still playing with dolls, even though exactly what age you were is forgotten. A trivial point, perhaps.

You followed through for (because of) your father. You were self-sustaining and raised your children alone. After you divorced your husband, you did not allow your family to fall apart or to become poor. You are their mother. Your children went to college.

You write for you now; you've been told it will slow things down. Maybe writing organizes your memories and makes them permanent such that they won't be lost once they are forgotten. You write stories that are true life. You write stories about your family, your life.

"They take me around with them. Like a baby – that's how I feel sometimes." Just once did you allude to a feeling of having given something up, of having left behind a life in Virginia for one that could not be yours in Michigan? Just once.

Would you write about your illness? "Yes, but I think it would be the last thing I write about." Which is interesting since dementia is a disease of memory and of personality. In saving your illness for last, your spirit is portrayed. A spark of a taunt, teasing dementia, saying that you will still be able to write your story.

You write for you now; you've been told it will slow things down.

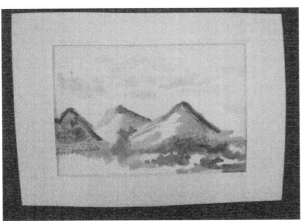

Sarah Williams, a second-year medical student, creatively helped a member of a memory loss program recall his past while she contemplates her role as a student doctor.

EVERYWHERE'S A MOUNTAIN

Sarah Williams

Where have we been, and where are we going? Often times we're headed there together.

The memory center welcomes you with an older, sweet receptionist seated by the door. The way she looks at you, inviting but slightly concerned behind her glasses, you begin to worry that she might be one of the many patients here hoping to regain something of their past. Then you wonder if it's about regaining the past so much as it is about gaining something of the future. Holding on to memories is a skill we need to move forward, strangely enough. The patients come here for help. So looking at the receptionist you worry that she might not be able to answer the question "Where should we go?" as you stand there in your untrained medical student place. The clothes don't quite fit yet.

But she offers you coffee, and this is just fine. Then she offers you a seat somewhere, and this is also fine, although everywhere the vinyl seat covers are worn through to the cloth. There are white fabric runs showing through the teal. Not spared the recession, you think, or maybe not so much money for keeping old memories alive. Maybe you have it wrong about money, and it's all about how many have sat here before you.

Eventually, you're brought to a room where a small man is standing next to a file cabinet rearranging a set of paper maché bowls that could otherwise be mistaken for paper maché eggs, broken across their egg middles and colored red, blue and white. He smiles like you've caught him in the act. A trick being played on the room's owner.

You meet the man. Thomas Frederick Curtis III. He tells you he's from "West by God Virginia," which is to say West Virginia. Although things are getting harder and harder for him to keep straight, he never forgets to add "By Gawd!" to his West Virginias, naked of their holy shroud. You've never heard of "West By God Virginia," and he tells you the name is from the state's secession from Virginia. From West Virginia being carved off from a piece of Virginia like God with a wood knife, deciding to save a good part. By God, and just in time. The old rot log was left behind.

And the way he describes West Virginia you imagine something crafted by God in his early days. "Everywhere there's a mountain," he tells you. Green trees, choking scrub growth. Up, up, or down, down; up and down, depending on how things are seen. Life perpetually fights on the slant, everything threatening to roll away and onward, no rock or root or foot spared that one force.

Thomas was born the youngest of twelve with a view of perpetual mountains. For his mother, you want to imagine a grade so steep to the house's foundation, the marriage bed, that the little boy just fell out of her, easy as gravity into her arms. Elsewhere, and slightly preceding this birth, a young woman labored in a different fold of the green valley blanket. She fell in love with a rich man visiting a resort in Jackson's Mill. Then he left, and she saw only mountains where his beautiful head had once been. She took to imagining that beautiful head still, hovering there in her arms like her baby was. Soon it didn't take much imagination at all.

"He had a Henry Ford face!" Thomas the third explains to you, when you're confused by his only living sister having been married to Henry Ford. Henry Ford's beautiful, unmarried mother gave him the name.

As for Thomas the third, he grew against gravity, learned from strong men. He helped his dad "cut filth" along the hillsides, keeping the pastures tidy of scrub growth and green debris. Some filth was hay, grown for the horses and cows, although there was more and more of a certain kind of animal that carried plenty of men and didn't need hay at all. One day Thomas's father was driving a load of hay into town when a pack surrounded him. The automobiles zoomed by so quickly they spooked his father's horse wagon and the whole hay load collapsed onto the man driving a swampstick pole right through his chest.

"He survived alright," Thomas tells you. "By God he was tough."

But with the spinning of those black wheels, the moment finally came where Thomas rolled away from the old mountain, not for lack of roots but for lack of work. He rolled toward the industry of Michigan, and you imagine him doing it with something of a smile, the way a bright copper penny could be mistaken for smiling, whirling along its edge in a penny funnel.

"My grandpa worked for GM," you tell Thomas, and he looks at you confused.

"What does that stand for?"

By the time you're finished saying "General Motors," there's a good smile on his face. Having taken up work at the Ford factory in Wixom and retiring there after 43 years, Thomas's old competitor has a place right next to "By God!" it seems. Loyalties to Ford and God are intact, just like they were forty years ago.

Of course he drove a Ford. He started out on the line and then worked his way up to supervisor, where he made good money and then retired. The union liked him, and he liked them. No problems there. A very nice story that he is still able to tell, but few are able to live these days in Michigan.

After saying your goodbye to Thomas, you think of what keeps memories around for good, or what waves a white handkerchief at them as if a boat were wanted to take them away. Make 'em drift by God!, onward and languidly away. You think of your grandfather, entirely unforgettable. You think of the many afternoons spent at his side and stories told and fondness for listening to others. Then you think about Thomas's winking moment, believing it would be easy to forget General Motors, having seen what you've seen. Chained factory gates. Old plants bogged down like wet shoeboxes that have windows to break. And those windows are broken all down the line of the building like so many failed chain links made of glass. The senior Henry Ford died. At some point later, the other Henry Ford died, leaving Thomas's sister behind. It's easy for you to forget what it once was. You never saw it the way Thomas saw it.

Now the time has come to leave the memory center. You're at the door, pausing, maybe wondering where you're off to next on this fall day. Those doctor clothes, those ideas for the future. Up and up? Down and down? A little of both, being the practical person that you are?

"Everywhere in Michigan is a mountain, sweetie," you half expect the receptionist to tell you, "Watch your step, and feel free to visit, anytime."

A Word about the U-M Supporting Programs

The **Cognitive Disorders Program** is a clinic within the Neurology Department at the University of Michigan Health System. Our group of neurologists, nurse practitioners, social workers, and neuropsychologists provides comprehensive, multi-disciplinary care to patients with cognitive impairment throughout their illness. We provide educational training to Residents in neurology, internal medicine, and psychiatry and to Fellows in geriatric medicine. We are located at the East Ann Arbor Health and Geriatrics Center, 4260 Plymouth Road, Ann Arbor, MI 48109. *For more information, please call (734) 764-6831, or visit www.uofmhealth.org/medical-services/dementia-and-alzheimers*

Established at the University of Michigan Health System and based in the Department of Neurology, the **Michigan Alzheimer's Disease Center** (MADC) aims to: a) conduct and support research on Alzheimer's disease and related disorders; b) promote state-of-the-art care for individuals experiencing memory loss or dementia; and c) enhance dementia awareness through collaborative education and outreach efforts. We are located at 2101 Commonwealth Blvd., Suite D., Ann Arbor, MI 48105. *To learn more about MADC related activities, please call (734) 936-8764 or visit www.med.umich.edu/alzheimers*

The **Silver Club Programs** are part of the Geriatrics Center's Social Work and Community Programs at the University of Michigan Health System. The Silver Club Programs, including **Coffeehouse, Mind Works, Elderberry Club, Wisdom Keepers** and the **Silver Club Enrichment Day Program** provide a safe, nurturing environment for older adults with mild to moderate memory loss. These programs are held at the Turner Senior Resource Center (TSRC). *To learn more about the Silver Club Programs offered at TSRC, please call 734-998-9352 or visit www.med.umich.edu /geriatrics/community/silverclub.htm*

Online Resources

Alzheimer's Association:
www.alz.org

Alzheimer's Disease Education and Referral Center:
www.nia.nih.gov/alzheimers

American Stroke Association:
www.strokeassociation.org

Family Caregiver Alliance:
www.caregiver.org

Lewy Body Dementia Association, Inc.:
www.lbda.org

National Parkinson Foundation:
www.parkinson.org

The Association for Frontotemporal Degeneration:
www.theaftd.org

Support Future Projects

This book was made possible by the generous donations from the **Michigan Alzheimer's Disease Center (MADC)** supporters. For information on supporting the MADC, **please call (734) 647-4178 or visit neurogiving@umich.edu**

Additional copies of this publication may be purchased from the MADC. **Please call (734) 936-8764 or email cassiem@umich.edu**

Proceeds from the sale of this book will be directed to future projects undertaken to support patients and families with memory loss.

THE EDITORS

Nan Barbas, MD, MSW, is the Director of the Cognitive Disorders Program, Department of Neurology, at the University of Michigan Health System.

Laura Rice-Oeschger, MA, LMSW, is the Wellness Coordinator at the Michigan Alzheimer's Disease Center and a consultant and facilitator at the U-M Silver Club Memory Loss Programs, a division of the U-M Geriatrics Center.

Cassie Starback, LMSW, is the Administrator for the Michigan Alzheimer's Disease Center, Department of Neurology, at the University of Michigan Health System.

19595520R00091

Made in the USA
Charleston, SC
02 June 2013